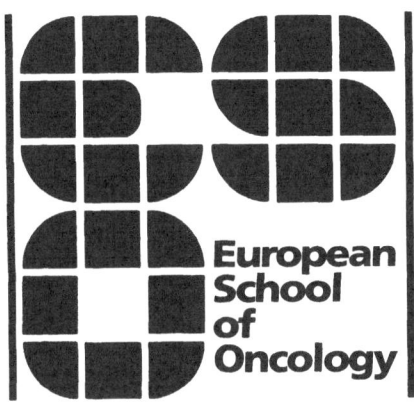

European
School
of
Oncology

Monographs

Series Editor: U. Veronesi

The European School of Oncology gratefully acknowledges sponsorship
for the Task Force received from AMGEN

Springer-Verlag
Berlin Heidelberg
GmbH

M. S. Aapro   D. Maraninchi   (Eds.)

The Role of Multiple Intensification in Medical Oncology

With 6 Figures and 16 Tables

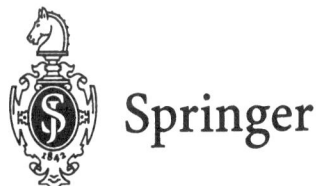

Springer

Dr. M. S. Aapro
Institut Multidisciplinaire d'Oncologie
1272 Genolier, Switzerland
and
European Institute of Oncology
Via Ripamonti 435
20141 Milano, Italy

Professor Dr. Maraninchi
Insitut Paoli Calmettes
232 Bd. de Sainte Marguerite
13273 Marseille Cedex 9, France

ISBN 978-3-662-01158-4   ISBN 978-3-662-01156-0 (eBook)
DOI 10.1007/978-3-662-01156-0

Library of Congress Cataloging-in-Publication Data
The role of multiple intensification in medical oncology: with 16 tables / [European School of Oncology].
M.S. Aapro; D. Maraninchi. - Berlin; Heidelberg; New York; Barcelona; Budapest; Hong Kong; London;
Milan; Paris; Santa Clara; Singapore; Tokyo: Springer 1998
  (Monographs / European School of Oncology)
  ISBN 978-3-662-01158-4

© Springer-Verlag Berlin Heidelberg 1998
Originally published by Springer-Verlag Berlin Heidelberg New York in 1998
Softcover reprint of the hardcover 1st edition 1998

Cover design: *design & production* GmbH, Heidelberg
Typesetting: Camera ready by editor
SPIN: 10132223   19/3133 - 5 4 3 2 1 0 – Printed on acid-free paper

Foreword

With this 40th volume we have come to the end of the ESO monograph series. The first volume was published 11 years ago and the series thus reflects the progress in oncology over a considerable period. With the advent of the era of electronic communication, this type of publication will increasingly compete with other means of dissemination of knowledge.

Therefore, apart from the continued publication of scientific updates in specific fields of oncological research, the editorial activities of the European School of Oncology will move into new directions. ESO launched its own dedicated online educational resource and information service on the Internet in the Spring of 1997, called Oncoweb. Another innovative project is the poduction of compact discs, the first volume of which is already available in a CD-I format, soon to be followed by a series of constantly updated educational material in new electronic formats, including CD-ROM.

The European School of Oncology wishes to thank all contributors over the years for their effort and commitment, the sponsoring companies for their trust and support, the publisher, Springer-Verlag, for the highly efficient and pleasant collaboration, and, last but not least, the readers for their interest and appreciation.

Umberto Veronesi
Chairman Scientific Committee
European School of Oncology

Contents

High Dose, Low Dose, No Dose: The Rights and Wrongs of Medical Oncology

Matti S. Aapro [1] and Dominique Maraninchi [2]

1   Institut Multidisciplinaire d'Oncologie, 1272 Genolier, Switzerland and Division of Medical Oncology, European Institute of Oncology, via Ripamonti 435, 20141 Milano, Italy
2   Institut Paoli-Calmettes, 232 Boulevard Sainte Marguerite, 13273 Marseille, France

The present volume is dedicated to various aspects of high-dose chemotherapy with progenitor cell support and the aim of the authors who have contributed to it is to highlight some of the more important areas under discussion, rather than to provide a complete overview of this expanding field of research. Such an endeavour would no doubt produce a little-read work, though one of some prestige. Why this choice, why not another?

Our attention has been focused on some of the ways in which resistance can be overcome, as it has been recognised that, whereas in any area of medical treatment an adequate dose is essential for a positive outcome, the results of high-dose therapy on obviously chemoresistant cancers have been mixed. The economic aspects of high-dose treatment with cellular support are currently under discussion and though, undoubtedly, such debates are important at the present time, they will be less so once the right indications have been established and patients will be cured or significantly palliated by these techniques.

The pharmacology of cytotoxic agents is modified by this type of high-dose chemotherapy and in order to develop the most rational regimens these changes must be identified. What is a rational regimen however?

Several approaches are illustrated in this volume and diverse outstanding results have been obtained with some single high-dose therapies and multiple high-dose treatments. Many questions remain unanswered in this exciting field and with the discovery of new, highly efficacious drugs, ongoing and future research must continue to address open issues, including:

* correct selection of patients to receive ablative high-dose chemotherapy supported with haematopoietic transplant;
* the role of non-ablative regimens, each drug delivered at the correct dose and schedule;
* the pharmacokinetic rationale of optimal combination of new and old drugs together and correct sequencing of their administration.

There would be no discussion, however, without growth factors, which play a key role in all these approaches. Moreover, the question is not solely whether to administer high-dose treatment or not, but it is about administering the most appropriate dose to achieve the best outcome, or even no dose at all in the case of truly chemotherapy-resistant tumours.

Haematological Support: Progenitor Cell Collection and Processing

Giovanni Martinelli [1], Fedro Peccatori [1] and Alessandro Massimo Gianni [2]

1   Division of Medical Oncology, European Institute of Oncology, Via Ripamonti 435, 20141 Milano
2   Division of Medical Oncology, Bone Marrow Transplant Unit, National Cancer Institute, Via Venezian 1, 20133 Milano, Italy

There is considerable interest in the use of peripheral blood progenitor cells (PBPC) for autografting patients with haematological and other malignancies. This interest is justified by the fact that PBPC transplant after high-dose chemotherapy (HDCT) results in more rapid haematological recovery, less morbidity, fewer platelet transfusions and lower hospitalisation costs.

The first clear evidence that peripheral blood progenitor cells could induce myeloid engraftment was obtained in 1959 when Marwin showed that the circulating blood cells of irradiated mice transfused with leukaphered blood were similar to the donor cells [1]. In 1962 Goodman and Hodgson demonstrated that erythrocytes, granulocytes and lymphocytes in the blood of recipient animals after infusion of homologous blood cells were donor in origin [2]. Since 1978 progenitor cells capable of engrafting an irradiated host have been demonstrated in several animal models such as guinea pigs [3], dogs [4], rhesus monkeys [5] and baboons [6].

Progenitor cells are fewer in the blood than in marrow. If we need 3×10^4 of fresh marrow cells to protect 50% of sublethally irradiated mice and induce 10 colony forming unit spleen cells (CFU), we need at least 100 times more blood leukocytes to induce the same number of CFUs [7].

Cytogenetic studies following allogeneic blood progenitor cell transplantation have led to the conclusion that under transplant conditions blood-derived progenitor cells are qualitatively equivalent to marrow-derived progenitor cells [8].

What is a Haematopoietic Progenitor Cell?

Definitions of haematopoietic progenitor cells vary according to the context in which they are considered. The exact nature of the cells that contribute to haematopoietic reconstitution is unknown.

The most stringent definition is based on the assumption that all haematopoietic cell differentiating steps are irreversible and hence the ultimate haematopoietic progenitor cell population is one whose members will regenerate and sustain long-term production of all other cells of the system [9]. The possibility to isolate progenitor cells has been hampered by the lack of specific assays. Early attempts to purify progenitor cells utilised density gradient separation or elutriation of mononuclear cells [10-12]. More recently, the observation that a monoclonal antibody raised against the leukaemia cell line KG-1A also reacts with some mononuclear progenitor cells in human bone marrow that differentiated into haematopoietic colonies, implemented an easier and faster method for the isolation of progenitor cells from other mononuclear cells [13]. The antigen recognised by this antibody was defined as CD34.

Berenson et al. in 1988 demonstrated that in sublethally irradiated primates, CD34+ cells were the cells necessary and sufficient for haematopoietic reconstitution [14]. Bernstein et al. in 1991 observed that CD34+ cells in bone marrow are heterogeneous, only a few of them being capable of self-renewal [15].

Several studies have demonstrated the existence of CD34+ cells devoid of other cell surface antigens. These studies defined these cells as "lineage negative" (lin-) cells, or cells that are in G0 or resistant to 5-FU [16-18].

These cells, however, under appropriate stimulation using preformed stromal layers or combination of cytokines, can give rise to multilineage colonies.

Progenitor Cell Isolation

The most widely used device for progenitor cell separation is the fluorescence activated cell sorter (FACS) that directly sorts cells labelled with an anti-CD34 antibody from T and B CD34+, lin- cells. Indeed FACS has the capability of providing homogeneous cells for a given antigen specificity. The limited amount of cells processed by FACS reduces its utility for cell separation for *in vitro* or small animal studies [16-18].

Immunomagnetic beads have been the alternative approach for the separation of certain cell subsets from marrow [19]. One or more antibodies of the same isotypes are incubated with the cells. Then, immunomagnetic microbeads coated with an isotype-specific anti-globulin are mixed and positive cells linked to the microbeads are separated using a strong magnetic field. Microbead-linked cells are then divided from unbound magnetic beads and from all other cells. Several groups have been successfully using this approach for *in vitro* and animal studies and, more recently, also for humans [19].

Bensiger et al. have used an avidin-biotin immunoabsorption column for progenitor cell isolation. This technique utilises the very high af-

Table 1. Increase in CFU-GM during GF administration*

Level of CFU-GM/ml (range)	
Pretreatment	Day 4 of GF administration
72 (15-150)	783 (144-5000)

* data from [21] and [22]

finity between the protein avidin and the vitamin biotin. Avidin is covalently linked to polyacrylamide beads which are sterilised and placed into plastic or glass columns. After incubation with anti-CD34 antibody, the marrow buffy coat is washed and incubated with a secondary biotinilated antibody. The labelled cells are then passed through the avidin column and repeatedly washed. Adherent cells are removed by gentle shaking. With the use of this method 13 patients were reinfused following high-dose chemotherapy and all patients had complete haematopoietic reconstitution. Further studies are warranted to appraise the clinical impact of these manipulations and the cost-benefit of the entire procedure [20].

Growth Factors (GF) and Peripheral Blood Progenitor Cells (PBPC)

Both G-CSF [21] and GM-CSF [22] administration increases the number of progenitor cells circulating in the peripheral blood (Table 1).

Table 2. PBPC mobilisation by myelosuppressive chemotherapy

Diseases	Chemotheraphy protocols
Acute myeloid leukaemia	TAD-like regimens
Chronic myeloid leukaemia	High-dose cyclophosphamide
Acute lymphoblastic leukaemia	IMPV 16
Non-Hodgkin's lymphomas	High-dose melphalan
Multiple myeloma	High-dose cyclophosphamide, vincristine, adriamycin, methylprednisolone
Ovarian cancer, breast cancer	High-dose cyclophosphamide
Paediatric neoplasms	Vincristine
	Adriamycin
	Daunorubicin
	Ara-c
	VP-16
	Cyclophosphamide

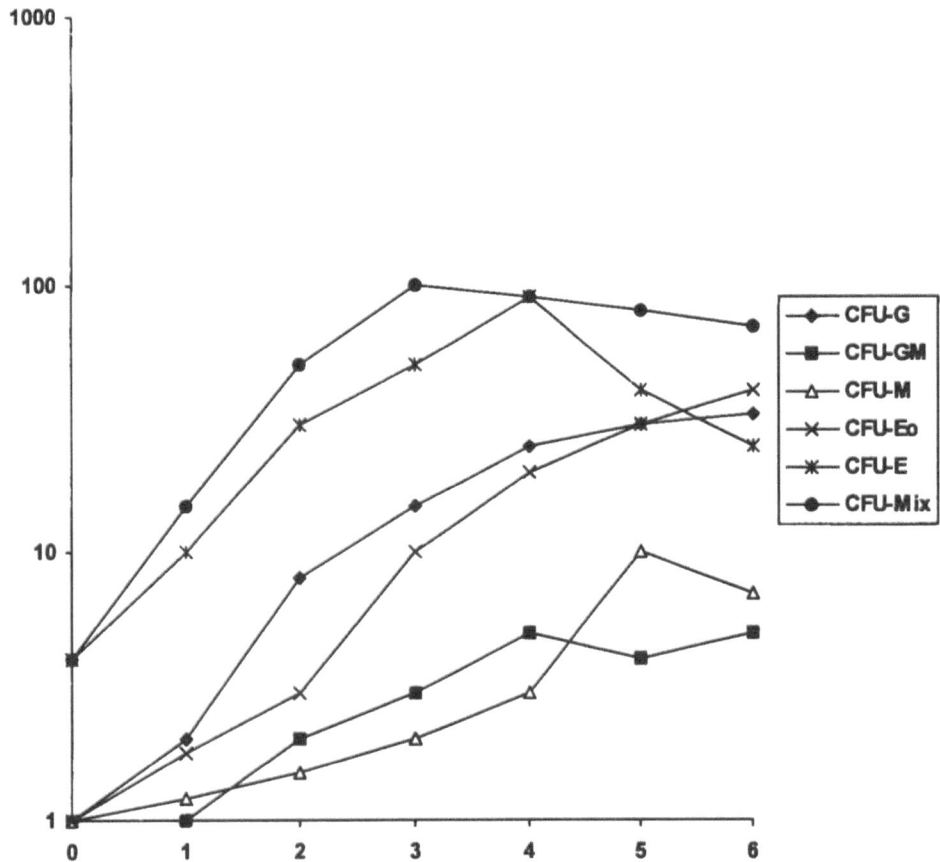

Fig. 1. Increase in circulating progenitor cells after GF administration (days 1-5). X-axis: days; y-axis: number of CFUx10^5

The use of growth factors results in an 8 to 100-fold increase in the number of progenitor cells and the magnitude of this rise is sufficient for harvesting enough progenitor cells for bone marrow reconstitution and transplantation (Fig. 1).

Peripheral Blood Progenitor Cells After Chemotherapy and Growth Factors

Progenitor cell mobilisation by myelosuppressive chemotherapy has been used in a large number of chemosensitive malignancies (Table 2). The magnitude of the rebound PBPC increase appears to be related to the intensity of the preceding myelosuppression and to the chemotherapy regimen used [23-26]. The use of colony stimulating factors during recovery from myelotoxic chemotherapy results in amplification of the mobilising effects induced by chemotherapy alone [25]. High-dose cyclophosphamide (HD CTX) (4-7 g/m^2) has been the most extensively studied mobilising regi-

men. It has the advantage that alkylating agents seem to spare the progenitor cells and are active against most lymphomas and solid tumours.

Cyclophosphamide administration is associated with brief but profound cytopenia, creating a potent stimulus to haematopoiesis. When HD CTX was combined with GM-CSF, the mean concentration of progenitor cells increased approximately 100-fold, allowing the harvesting of more than 30 x 10^4 CFU-GM/kg body weight [26].

The same results have been obtained when G-CSF or other cytokines were used after HD CTX [27]. This very high yield required only 2 or 3 leukaphereses on consecutive days. The rise in circulating progenitor cell number after high-dose CTX occurs during the recovery phase of peripheral blood neutrophil and platelet counts and is of brief duration. For these reasons it is critical to carefully choose the time when peripheral blood progenitor cells must be collected on the basis of easy and reproducible parameters. These parameters must be simple,

Table 3. CFU-GM levels in relation to peripheral blood leukocyte counts (n=28)*

Leukocyte counts (x 10^9/L)	1.0	1.5	2.0	3.0	4.0
Mean CFU-GM (x 10^3/L)	1338	1172	2025	2572	3193

*modified from [36]

quick and predictive. CFU-GM assaying predicts the number of circulating progenitor cells in the peripheral blood but needs 14 days to yield results. On the basis of retrospective analysis correlating changes in blood counts with CFU-GM levels, many laboratories have designed protocols to establish the exact period for PBPC harvest based on blood values. The majority of these protocols consider leukapheresis when leukocyte counts reach 1.5 x 10^6/L or when mononuclear cells reach 3.0 x 10^8/kg body weight (Table 3). However, the problem may be overcome by the adoption of simpler, more reproducible assays for progenitor cells, such as the phenotypic analysis of CD34+ cells using direct flow cytometry of whole blood [28-30].

Colony Stimulating Factors Without Chemotherapy

Both G-CSF [29,31] and GM-CSF [30,32] can be used alone to mobilise large numbers of progenitor cells which can be successfully reinfused in the autograft setting to provide leukocyte, haemoglobin and platelet recovery after HD chemotherapy. Growth factors are used alone for 6-7 days at dosages ranging from 10 µg/kg daily to 12 µg/kg daily with leukapheresis being performed on day 5, 6 or 7.

The results of progenitor cell mobilisation with growth factors alone are consistent, even if there is no randomised study comparing GF ± CT. GF + CT could yield more progenitor cells than GF without CT but this procedure would be inappropriate in healthy allograft donors.

Collection of Blood Progenitor Cells

The technology of peripheral blood progenitor cell collection is a by-product of the expertise in extracorporeal blood component separation.

By the early 1980s microprocessor-controlled, menu-driven automated blood cell separators were capable of efficiently separating whole blood into granulocytes, mononuclear cells, platelets and plasma in a closed continuous flow system. Meanwhile it was shown that the primitive haematopoietic progenitor cell in peripheral blood co-separated with lymphocytes and monocytes on density gradients and haematopoietic reconstitution could be achieved with these blood progenitor cells [33].

Table 4. Comparison of different cell separators

	Haemonetics	Baxter CS3000+	CobeSpectra
Number of procedures	41	25	60
Median blood volumes	4.4	9.2	9.1
MNC collecting efficiency %	43	53	47
CFU-GM collecting efficiency %	63	103	83
Volume final product (ml)	424	50	98

Collecting efficiency: $$\frac{\text{absolute cell count in the concentrate (cells) x 100}}{\text{cell count (cells/ml) x total volume processed (ml)}}$$

Haemonetics V30 and Baxter Fenwal CS 3000+ were the first blood cell separators used. Currently CS3000+ and Cobe Spectra are the two most commonly used separators. They separate in a closed continuous flow circuit, are easy to operate and produce less circulating disturbance than the older separators. Another advantage is that the lesser volume of the final product corresponds to a higher efficiency in CFU-GM collection (Table 4).

All these machines can safely operate with peripheral veins, although previous cytotoxic damage to the venous tree may dictate the use of other approaches such as subclavicular silicon rubber catheters (Hickman's catheter).

Side effects with continuous blood flow separation are uncommon. Citrate overdose and boredom can be relieved by a glass of calcium gluconate and friendly apheresis staff. Catheter obstruction is uncommon and can be resolved by flushing with heparinised solution or bolus injection of urokinase.

During steady-phase haematopoiesis haemoglobin and platelet counts may drop following apheresis [34]. In the recovery phase leukocyte and lymphocyte counts may also diminish, but this is rarely clinically significant [35].

REFERENCES

1   Marwin RM: Repopulation of hematopoietic tissues of x-irradiated mice by cells from leukemoid blood. Proc Soc Exp Biol Med 1959 (101):9-11
2   Goodman JW and Hodgson BS: Evidence for stem cells in peripheral blood of mice. Blood 1962 (19): 702-704
3   Malinin TI, Perry VP, Kerby CC et al: Peripheral leukocyte infusion into lethally irradiated guinea pigs. Blood 1965 (25):693-702
4   Cavins JA, Scheer SC, Thomas ED et al: The recovery of lethally irradiated dogs given infusions of autologous leukocytes preserved at -80° C. Blood 1964 (23):38-43
5   Storb R, Prentice R, Thomas ED: Letter. N Engl J Med 1977 (297):58
6   Storb R, Graham TC, Epstein RB et al: Demonstration of haemopoietic stem cells in the peripheral blood of baboons by cross circulation. Blood 1977 (50):537-542
7   Lewis JR and Trobaugh FE Jr: The assay to the transplantation potential of fresh and stored bone marrow by two in vivo systems. Am Acad Sci NY 1964 (114):677
8   Carbonell F, Calvo W, Fliedner M et al: Cytogenetic studies in dogs after total body irradiation and allogeneic transfusion with cryopreserved blood mononuclear cells: observation in long term chimeras. Int J Cell Cloning 1984 (2):81-88
9   Eavis CJ and Eavis AC: Stem and progenitor cells in the blood. In: Gale RP, Juttner C, Henon P (eds) Blood Stem Cell Transplants. Cambridge University Press 1994 pp 20-21
10 Visser JWM and Bol SJL: A two step procedure for obtaining 80 fold enriched suspensions of murine plenipotent hemopoietic stem cells. Stem Cells 1981 (1):240-249
11 Ellis WM, Georgiov GM, Roberton DM et al: The use of discontinuous percoll gradients to separate population of cells from human bone marrow and peripheral blood. J Immunol Methods 1984 (66):9-16
12 De Witte T, Hoogenhout J, De Pauw B et al: Depletion of donor lymphocytes by counterflow centrifugation successfully prevents acute graft versus host disease in matched allogenic marrow transplantation. Blood 1986 (67):1302-1308
13 Civin CI, Strauss LC, Brovall C et al: Antigenic analysis of haematopoiesis. An hematopoietic progenitor cell surface antigen defined by a monoclonal antibody raised against KG-1a cells. J Immunol 1984 (1335):157-165
14 Berenson RJ, Andrews RG, Bensinger WI et al: Antigen CD34+ marrow cells engraft lethally irradiated baboons. J Clin Invest 1988 (81):951-955
15 Bernstein ID, Andrews RT, Zsebo KM et al: Recombinant human stem cell factor enhances the formation of colonies by CD34+ and CD34+lin- cells, and the generation of colony forming cells cultured with interleukin 3 (IL-3), granulocyte macrophage colony stimulating factor (GM-CSF), or granulocyte colony stimulating factor (G-CSF). Blood 1991 (77): 2316-2321
16 Andrews RG, Singer JW, Bernstein ID: Human hematopoietic precursors in long term culture: single CD34+ cells that lack detectable T, B, and myeloid antigens produce multiple colony-forming cells when cultured with marrow stromal cells. J Exp Med 1990 (172):355-358
17 Srour EF, Brandt JE, Briddell RA et al: Human D34+ HLA-DR bone marrow cells contain progenitor cells capable of self renewal multilineage differentiation and long term in vitro hematopoiesis. Blood Cells 1991 (17):287-295
18 Terstappen LWMN, Huang S, Safford M et al: Sequential generations of hematopoietic colonies derived from single monolineage committed CD34+ CD38- progenitor cells. Blood 1991 (77):1218-1227
19 Wormmcester J, Stiekema F, De Groot C et al: Immunoselective cell separation. Methods Enzymol 1990 (184): 314-319
20 Bensinger WI, Berenson RJ, Andrews RG et al: Engrafting after infusion of CD34 enriched marrow cells. Int J Cell Cloning 1992 (10 Suppl 1):35-37
21 Durhsen U, Villeval JI, Boyd J et al: Effects of recombinant granulocyte colony stimulating factor on hematopoietic progenitor cells in cancer patients. Blood 1988 (72):2074-2081
22 Socinski MA, Cannistra SA, Elins A et al: Granulocyte-macrophage colony stimulating factor expands the circulating haemopoietic progenitor cell compartment in man. Lancet 1988 (1):1194-1198
23 To LB, Haylock DN, Kimber RJ et al: High levels of circulating haematopoietic stem cells in very early remission from acute non lymphoblastic leukemia and their collection and cryopreservation. Br J Haematol 1984 (58):399-410
24 To LB, Shepperd KM, Haylock DN et al: Single high dose of cyclophosphamide enables the collection of high numbers of haemopoietic stem cells from the peripheral blood. Exp Hematol 1990 (18):442-447
25 Reiffers J, Bernard KM, Marit G et al: Collection of blood derived hematopoietic stem cells and application for autologous transplantation. Bone Marow Transplant 1984 (1):371-372
26 Gianni AM, Siena S, Bregni M et al: Granulocyte-macrophage colony-stimulating factor to harvest circulating haematopoietic stem cells for autotransplantation. Lancet 1989 (ii):580-585
27 Gianni AM, Siena S, Bregni M et al: Very rapid and complete haematopoietic reconstitution following myeloablative treatments: the role of circulating stem cells harvested after high-dose cylophosphamide and GM-CSF. In: Dicke KA, Spitzer G, Jagamath S, Evinger Hodges MJ (eds) Autologous Bone Marrow Transplantation. 4th ed. The University of Texas Press, Houston 1994 pp 723-731
28 Gianni AM, Bregni M, Siena S et al: Clinical usefulness and optimal harvesting of peripheral blood stem cells mobilized by high dose cyclophosphamide and R GM-CSF. In: Wunder EW, Henon PR (eds) Peripheral Blood Stem Cell Autografts. Springer Verlag, Heidelberg 1993 pp 145-154
29 Pettengel R, Demuynck H, Testa NG et al: The engraftment capacity of peripheral blood stem cells (PBSC) mobilized with chemotherapy +/- G-CSF. Int J Cell Cloning 1992 (10 Suppl 1):59-61
30 Siena S, Bregni M, Brando B et al: Flow cytometry for clinical estimation of circulating hematopoietic

progenitors. Blood 1991 (77):138-147

31 Sheridan WP, Begley CG, Juttner CA et al: Effect of peripheral blood progenitor cells mobilized by filgrastim (G-CSF) on platelet recovery after high-dose chemotherapy. Lancet 1992 (339):640-644

32 Elias A, Mazanet R, Anderson K et al: GM-CSF mobilized peripheral blood stem cell autografts - the DFCI/BIH experience. Int J Cell Cloning 1992 (10 Suppl 1):149-151

33 Juttner CA, To LB, Haylock DN et al: Circulating autologous stem cells collected from acute man lymphoblastic leukemia produce prompt incomplete haemopoietic reconstitution after high-dose melphalan or sublethal chemoradiotherapy. Br J Haematol 1985 (61):739-746

34 Korbling M, Fliedner TM, Pfeliger H et al: Collection of large quantities of granulocytes-macrophage progenitor cells (CFUs) in man by continuous flow leukapheresis. Scand J Haematol 1980 (24):22-28

35 Haylock DN, Canty A, Throp D et al: A discrepancy between the instantaneous and the overall collection efficiency of the Fenwal CS 3000 for peripheral blood stem cell apheresis. J Clin Apheresis 1992 (7):6-11

36 To LB and Juttner CA: Stem cell mobilization by myelosuppressive chemotherapy. In: Wunder EW, Henon PR (eds) Peripheral Blood Stem Cell Autografts. Springer Verlag, Heidelberg 1993 pp 132-144

Pharmacotoxicology of High-Dose Thiotepa

Gilles Vassal and Olivier Hartmann

Paediatric Department, Institut Gustave-Roussy, Rue Camille Desmoulins, 94805 Villejuif, France

Thiotepa is an alkylating agent that was first synthesised in the 1950s. It can be administered intravenously, intravesically and intrathecally. At conventional doses the main adverse effect is haematopoietic toxicity. For about 10 years now thiotepa has been used at high doses prior to bone marrow transplantation. High-dose thiotepa has been particularly developed in the USA, while high-dose melphalan is preferred in Europe.

Mechanism of Action and Biotransformation

The alkylating properties of thiotepa are due to its aziridine functions. At physiological temperature and pH, chemical or enzymatic hydrolysis of thiotepa and its metabolite, tepa, releases aziridine, a highly reactive monofunctional alkylating agent. Aziridine reacts with guanine or adenine to form mono-adducts on one of the two DNA strands. Accumulation of these lesions causes cell death. Thiotepa is considered as a stable and lipophilic form of aziridine, for which it serves as a carrier to penetrate inside the cell [3]. At high concentrations thiotepa (but not tepa) directly damages DNA by forming inter-strand bridges.

Thiotepa is transformed into tepa, its active metabolite, by the cytochrome P450 system. The liver being the richest organ in cytochrome P450, it is the main site of thiotepa metabolism. The human cytochrome P450s involved in hepatic biotransformation of thiotepa have not yet been identified.

Thiotepa and tepa are conjugated to glutathion and thereby form inactive metabolites. This results in a transient depletion of intracellular glutathion, a phenomenon also observed with other anticancer drugs such as cyclophosphamide. Conjugation to glutathion can participate in mechanisms of resistance to thiotepa in malignant cells. Intracellular glutathion depletion (by specific drugs or other anticancer agents) can sensitise cells to the cytotoxic action of thiotepa. Therapeutic synergy is thus expected with the cyclophosphamide-thiotepa combination, among others [11].

Maximum Tolerated Doses

The maximum tolerated dose of thiotepa without haematopoietic support has recently been reassessed in adults and children [5,9]. It is 65 mg/m^2 as a short injection or lengthy infusion every 3 to 4 weeks. Use of haematopoietic growth factors does not allow the dose to be increased beyond 75 mg/m^2 because of cumulative platelet toxicity. At conventional doses, myelosuppression is the dose-limiting form of toxicity.

The maximum tolerated dose of thiotepa monotherapy with haematopoietic progenitor cell support is 900 mg/m^2 [12]. Thiotepa is usually administered at a dose of 300 mg/m^2/day, either in 3 short infusions (30 to 60 minutes) or continuously. At high doses neurotoxicity is the dose-limiting form of toxicity.

Pharmacology of Thiotepa

Thiotepa and tepa are assayed in biological fluids by means of gas chromatography. The pharmacokinetics of thiotepa has been described after intravenous administration of conventional doses (12 to 75 mg/m^2) as a bolus or an infusion (2 to 8 hours), and after high doses followed by bone marrow transplantation (135 to 405 mg/m^2/day, as a bolus, short infusion or continuous infusion).

Plasma concentrations generally follow a biexponential curve, with a mean α half-life of 6 to 21 minutes and a mean β half-life of 1.3 to 4 hours. Tepa, the main metabolite, appears rapidly in the plasma after intravenous administration of thiotepa. Its half-life of elimination is longer (4 to 15 hours).

The pharmacokinetics of thiotepa is not linear. Average total plasma clearance falls in adults and children when the dose increases from 30 to 75 mg/m^2. This phenomenon is attributed to saturation of thiotepa biotransformation into tepa. After administration of high doses (135 to 405 mg/m^2), the plasma clearance of thiotepa is comparable to that observed at the highest conventional doses (75 mg/m^2) [6,8]. During simultaneous administration of high doses of thiotepa and cyclophosphamide as a continuous infusion lasting 96 hours, thiotepa clearance increases with time, due either to auto-induction of thiotepa metabolism or an interaction with cyclophosphamide [6].

The level of protein binding in plasma, measured by steady-state dialysis, is only about 10%.

Thiotepa clearance is mainly extra-renal. Only 1.5% of the dose administered (12 mg/m^2) is eliminated in urine during the following 12 hours. At the same time, 4% of the dose is eliminated in the form of thiotepa and 23% in the form of unidentified alkylating molecules (alkylating activity measured with paranitrobenzylpyridine) [2]. Thiotepa is largely metabolised by the liver, potentially creating a risk of drug interactions, especially with drugs that induce or inhibit hepatic enzymes (e.g. anticonvulsants). No interactions have been reported to date, but thiotepa should not be coadministered with drugs influencing hepatic metabolism, whenever possible.

Thiotepa and tepa penetrate into the central nervous system [5]. Equivalent concentrations are present in plasma and cerebrospinal fluid from 1 to 8 hours after the end of the infusion.

Toxicity of High-Dose Thiotepa

Wolff reviewed phase I trials of high-dose thiotepa monotherapy (135 to 1575 mg/m^2) followed by bone marrow transplantation [12]. The main forms of extra-haematopoietic toxicity were neurological, gastrointestinal, cutaneous and hepatic.

Haematopoietic Toxicity

Neutropenia and thrombocytopenia occur 7 to 10 days after treatment. Haematopoietic reconstitution takes 2 to 3 weeks on average (more than 1 month in 20% of patients in these phase I trials). Persistent thrombocytopenia is observed in 5% of patients receiving doses above 405 mg/m^2. Beyond 180 mg/m^2, the pattern and severity of haematopoietic toxicity remain fairly uniform.

Neurological Toxicity

Central neurological toxicity manifests itself in the form of headache, altered consciousness (confusion, amnesia, drowsiness, hallucinations, etc.) and behaviour disorders. Life-threatening convulsive states and coma have been reported at doses above 1 g/m^2 [8]. The neurotoxicity of thiotepa is dose-dependent and dose-limiting. At the maximum tolerated dose of 900 mg/m^2, moderate and reversible neurological signs are observed in 5% of cases.

Gastrointestinal Toxicity

Nausea and vomiting are frequent, but are moderate and easily controlled with standard antiemetics. Lesions of the gastrointestinal mucosa, with mucositis, oesophagitis and, in some cases, enterocolitis, are frequent and dose dependent. This type of toxicity is similar to that observed with melphalan. It is severe beyond 900 mg/m^2. It can be potentiated by coadministration of other agents damaging the gastrointestinal mucosa.

Cutaneous Toxicity

This involves an occasional maculopapular rash of the palms and soles, leading to desquamation, but can also be more diffuse. As with many alkylating agents given at high doses, hyperpigmentation predominating in the skin folds and genitalia is frequent, and can persist for several months.

Hepatic Toxicity

The only manifestation in most cases is isolated, transient hepatic cytolysis, sometimes associated with hyperbilirubinaemia. No cases of hepatic veno-occlusive disease have been reported after high-dose thiotepa monotherapy.

Antitumoural Activity

In the course of these phase I trials, which involved 217 patients with various tumour types, Wolff calculated that the rate of complete and partial responses was 50%. The main histological forms sensitive to high-dose thiotepa are adenocarcinomas of the breast, ovary and lung, malignant melanoma, glioblastoma, germ cell tumours, neuroblastoma, and soft-tissue sarcomas [12].

Thiotepa in High-Dose Chemotherapy Protocols

Thiotepa is currently included in high-dose chemotherapy protocols used to treat breast and brain tumours. The cyclophosphamide-thiotepa combination has been developed at the Dana Farber Institute in Boston. The 3-drug combination cyclophosphamide-thiotepa-carboplatin (CTC) has become a standard high-dose protocol for breast cancer [1]. One particularity of this protocol is that the three drugs are administered as a continuous infusion. The excellent distribution of thiotepa in the central nervous system has led to its inclusion in experimental protocols for brain tumours such as

etoposide-thiotepa (malignant glial tumours) [4] and busulfan-thiotepa (childhood medulloblastomas) [7]. Other combinations are being tested in haematological malignancies [10].

REFERENCES

1 Ayash U, Elias A, Wheeler C et al: Double dose-intensive chemotherapy with autologous marrow and peripheral-blood progenitor-cell support for metastatic breast cancer: a feasibility study. J Clin Oncol 1994 (12):37-44
2 Cohen BE, Egorin MJ, Kohlhepp EA, Aisner J, Gutierrez PL: Human pharmacokinetics and urinary excretion of thiotepa and its metabolites. Cancer Treat Rep 1986 (70):859-864
3 Egorin MJ, Snyder SW, Pan S, Daly C: Cellular transport and accumulation of thiotepa. Semin Oncol 1990 (17 suppl 3):7-17
4 Finlay JL, August C, Packer R et al: High-dose multiagent chemotherapy followed by bone marrow rescue for malignant astrocytomas of childhood and adolescence. J Neurol Oncol 1990 (9):239-248
5 Heidemann RL, Cole DE, Balis F: Phase I and pharmacokinetic evaluation of thiotepa in the cerebrospinal fluid and plasma of pediatric patients: evidence for dose-dependent plasma clearance of thiotepa. Cancer Res 1989 (49):736-741
6 Henner WD, Shea TC, Furlong EA et al: Pharmacokinetics of continuous infusion of high-dose thiothepa. Cancer Treat Rep 1987 (71):1043-1047
7 Kalifa C, Hartmann O, Demeocq F et al: High-dose busulfan and thiotepa with autologous bone marrow transplantation in childhood malignant brain tumors: a phase II study. Bone Marrow Transplant 1992 (9): 227-233
8 Lazarus HM, Reed MC, Spitzer TR, Rabas MS, Blumor JL: High-dose in thiotepa and cryopreserved autologous bone marrow transplantation for therapy of refractory cancer. Cancer Treat Rep 1987 (71): 689-695
9 O'Dwyer PJ, La Creta F, Engstrom PF: Phase I/pharmacokinetic reevaluation of thiotepa. Cancer Res 1991 (51):3171-3176
10 Przepiorka D, Ippoliti C, Giralt S et al: A phase II study of high-dose thiotepa, busulfan and cyclophosphamide as a preparative regimen for allogeneic transplantation. Bone Marrow Transplant 1994 (14):449-453
11 Teicher BA, Holden SA, Eder JP, Herman S, Antman K, Frei III E: Preclinical studies relating to the use of thiotepa in the high-dose setting alone and in combination. Semin Oncol 1990 (17 suppl 3):18-32
12 Wolff SN, Herzig RH, Fay JW: High-dose N,N',N''-triethylenethiophosphoramide (thiotepa) with autologous bone marrow transplantation: phase I studies. Sem Oncol 1990 (17 suppl 3):2-6

Pharmacotoxicology of High-Dose VP-16

Gilles Vassal and Olivier Hartmann

Paediatric Department, Institut Gustave-Roussy, Rue Camille Desmoulins, 94805 Villejuif, France

Two contrasting modes of VP-16 administration are currently under study: low doses by the oral route for long periods [13], and infusion of high doses combined with total body irradiation (TBI) or other chemotherapy regimens, prior to transplantation of autologous or allogeneic haematopoietic progenitor cells.

Mechanism of Action

VP-16 was long considered to damage the mitotic spindle, but this is not the case: VP-16 is in fact a specific inhibitor of DNA-topoisomerase II. It does not intercalate between DNA base pairs, contrary to other topoisomerase II inhibitors such as anthracyclines.

Topoisomerase II is a nuclear enzyme that creates temporary breaks in DNA, through which it passes another double-stranded section of DNA before repairing the break. It thus unravels DNA and contributes to the physiological balance required for DNA replication and transcription. It also plays an important role in chromatin structure by anchoring DNA loops to the nuclear matrix. It is involved in the assembly of chromatin, in the condensation and decondensation of chromosomes during the cell cycle, and in chromosome segregation during mitosis. The activity of topoisomerase II varies in the course of the cell cycle (increasing during the S, G2 and M phases).

VP-16 interacts with topoisomerase II and stabilises the cleavable complex formed by topoisomerase II and DNA. In this way it prevents the phase during which the cut ends are religated and the DNA-topoisomerase complex is dissociated. This stabilisation of the cleavable complex persists as long as topoisomerase II is exposed to sufficient concentrations of VP-16 in the nucleus. In other words, it is reversible when VP-16 is eliminated. The amount of damage is proportional to the quantity of topoisomerase present in the nucleus, the concentration of VP-16, and the time during which the enzyme is exposed to VP-16. Accumulation of such lesions is the first step in a cascade of events that lead to cell death; the latter include inhibition of DNA and RNA synthesis, an increased frequency of sister chromatid exchanges and chromosomal aberrations, and premitotic blockade in the S phase or the beginning of the G2 phase. This leads to a halt in cell cycling [7, 15].

VP-16 is therefore most active on cells undergoing DNA synthesis. Its cytotoxic action depends on its concentration and the exposure time. For a given exposure time there is a linear correlation between the dose and toxicity [7]. Experimental data obtained with leukaemic mice (L1210 and P388) have confirmed the importance of the dose and dosing schedule. The therapeutic action of VP-16 is more potent after multiple doses than after a single dose. In addition, dose fractionation allows the total dose to be increased [7].

These preclinical results suggest that dose increments and/or longer treatment periods would improve the therapeutic efficacy of VP-16 in the clinical setting. This warrants clinical trials of protocols involving high doses or lengthy oral administration. In addition, these data underline the importance of the dosing schedule during administration of high doses.

Maximum Tolerated Doses of VP-16

The first phase I trials were conducted in the late 1970s [7,8] with various dosing schedules. The conventional doses most often used were 300 to 500 mg/m^2, administered over a 3- to 5-day period every 3 to 4 weeks. Myelosuppression was considered dose-limiting, while little extra-haematopoietic toxicity was observed. Nevertheless, myelosuppression was moderate according to current criteria: fewer than 10% of patients had leukopenia below 1,000/mm^3, and thrombocytopenia (<50,000/ mm^3) was rare (mainly in patients with marrow involvement).

The moderate bone marrow toxicity, lack of extra-haematopoietic toxicity, and experimental data demonstrating a dose-dependent cytotoxic action led to phase I trials of high doses in the 1980s, with or without bone marrow transplantation [24,31]. The maximum tolerated dose of VP-16 monotherapy was 2.4 to 3.0 g/m^2, at which mucositis became the dose-limiting toxic effect.

Since then, high-dose VP-16 has been used in many types of conditioning regimens. A brief scan of the literature shows the extreme variety of high-dose VP-16 regimens in terms of:
- duration of treatment (1 to 3 days);
- duration of the infusion (30 minutes to 72 hours);
- preparation of VP-16 (dilutions of ≤0.4 mg/ml and 1 mg/ml; use of VP-16 undiluted);
- use of routine premedication.

All these parameters, as well as coadministered drugs, influence the maximum tolerated dose. Nonetheless, mucositis is still the main dose-limiting toxic effect. One of the most common regimens, especially in combination with total body irradiation, is the administration of 60 mg/kg as a 3- to 4-hour infusion [2], but several studies have suggested that slower infusion of high-dose VP-16 markedly reduces the severity of mucositis. For example, Brown reached a dose of 4.2 g/m^2 in combination with cyclophosphamide by using a fixed-rate continuous infusion [3], and Gianni observed very few cases of mucositis during infusion of 2.4 g/m^2 over 10 to 12 hours [10].

Modes of High-Dose VP-16 Administration

The instability of VP-16 in solution makes it difficult to administer high doses. The optimal mode depends on the duration of the infusion, the total dose to be infused and the fluid volume the patient can reasonably tolerate.

The instability of VP-16 solutions is shown by the appearance of whitish crystals in the infusion line. Stability depends on the concentration and time. At concentrations of 0.4 mg/ml and less, VP-16 is stable in 0.9% NaCl and 5% glucose for at least 8 hours at room temperature [18]. However, such a concentration implies very large amounts of fluid when high doses of VP-16 are used, especially when they are administered over periods of only 1 to 3 h. At concentrations of 1 mg/ml or more, crystals begin to form after 5 minutes with shaking and 30 minutes without shaking. Many teams administer VP-16 at a concentration of 1 mg/ml [1,11,31] and do not mention stability problems in their publications. Some, like Blume, state that they change flasks every hour during VP-16 infusions (1 mg/ml) lasting 4 hours [1]. More recent work has shown that VP-16 is stable for more than 8 hours at room temperature at concentrations of 10 mg/ml or more. The lower and upper concentration limits for VP-16 infusion are 0.4 mg/ml and 10 mg/ml.

In 1986, to overcome the problem of fluid volume and the excessive amounts of sodium delivered during high-dose VP-16 administration, Lazarus proposed using the injectable preparation undiluted (20 mg/ml) [20]. VP-16 was administered with a push-syringe, over 3 to 4 hours, with infusion equipment free of ABS plastics (acetonitrile, butadiene or styrene) that can split on contact with VP-16. This mode of administration (undiluted commercial preparation) was chosen by several teams, and the immediate toxicity varied from one report to another [9,10,21,22]. Schwinghammer [27] observed a higher frequency of hypotension, fever and anaphylactic reactions, which were rare in Mross' experience [23]. According to Gianni, tolerability was significantly improved by systemic steroids [10]. Given the numerous differences between teams it is impossible to establish the respective roles of the dilution, total dose and infusion rate in these phenomena. Recently, Mross conducted a pharmacokinetic study that demonstrated the bioequivalence of two modes of VP-16 administration (30 to 45 mg/kg over 6 hours) using either a 0.5 mg/ml solution in 0.9% NaCl (1 L/h) or the undiluted commercial preparation at 20 mg/ml [22]. Published data suggest that VP-16 can be administered undiluted, but that precautions must be taken (type of materials) and vital signs must be monitored closely.

Pharmacology of High-Dose VP-16

The VP-16 plasma concentration generally declines according to a two-compartment model, composed of a first rapid distribution phase (α half-life 30-60 min) and an elimination phase (β half-life 5-8 hours) [7,12,14,19,22,28]. The pharmacokinetics of VP-16 remains linear as the dose increases; in other words there is no saturation or induction of clearance. Mean plasma clearance is 20 to 30 ml/min/m^2, and 35% to 40% of the dose is eliminated unchanged in urine [14]. Biliary excretion in unchanged form is weak (0.9 to 2.1%) after conventional doses. The remainder of the dose is biotransformed into several metabolites, some of which are eliminated in urine (20% of the dose is eliminated in urine in the form of metabolites) [7].

Plasma Protein Binding

VP-16 binds avidly to plasma proteins (about 94%). The free fraction of VP-16 in plasma varies from 6% to 37% according to the patient. The free fraction is significantly larger in patients with hypoalbuminaemia or hyperbilirubinaemia [29].

Metabolism

Three types of metabolite have been identified in humans: hydroxyacids, the aglycone metabolite, and conjugation products [15]. Hydroxyacids and conjugation products, which are inactive, are eliminated in the bile and urine, where they account for approximately 20% of the dose. The aglycone metabolite, which is cytotoxic (inducing DNA strand breaks in the presence of topoisomerase II), has not been detected after conventional doses. The use of sensitive and specific analytical techniques (mass spectrometry) has revealed the presence of the aglycone metabolite in plasma at a concentration of 5 to 7 ng/ml 48 hours after administration of 350 mg/m^2/d x 5 [12]. This observation implies that bone marrow or peripheral progenitor cells should only be reinfused 72 hours after the last dose of VP-16.

Tissue Distribution

During administration of high doses, VP-16 is secreted in saliva at variable concentrations than can reach 25% of the corresponding plasma concentration [12]. This contributes to the mucosal toxicity of VP-16. VP-16 penetrates poorly into CSF, with reported concentrations of 0.1 to 2 µg/ml [15]. VP-16 is detectable in pleural effusions and ascitic fluid.

Effect of Dose Fractionation

Many teams have analyzed the plasma pharmacokinetics of VP-16 at various doses according to the mode of infusion (30 minutes to 72 hours). Increasing the duration of infusion reduces the peak concentration and prolongs exposure to weaker concentrations, without changing total systemic exposure (area under the concentration curve).
There have been no pharmacodynamic studies of the relation between the peak concentration and mucositis after high-dose monotherapy, and none formally demonstrating the value of continuous infusion. Nevertheless, the dose reached by Brown (4.2 g/m^2 during continuous infusion, compared to 60 mg/kg $\cong$ 2.4 g/m^2 over 4 hours conventionally) pleads in favour of continuous infusion [3].

Plasma Concentration at the Time of Transplantation

When bone marrow or peripheral progenitor cell allografting or autografting is envisaged, the presence of cytotoxic compounds at the time of reinfusion can reduce the chances of success. The risk is linked to the circulating concentration of VP-16, but also to that of its metabolites, such as the aglycone, which is present in plasma at cytotoxic concentrations for up to 48 hours after the end of treatment. Reported plasma concentrations of VP-16 at the time of transplantation are variable [22,23,26-28]. Concentrations of 0.3 to 0.5 µg/ml are considered to be harmless for the graft. While several teams have studied VP-16 concentrations at the time of grafting and their effect on the growth of bone marrow colonies *in vitro*, none has clearly established a link between plasma concentrations and the time required for haematopoietic recovery in the clinical setting. The accepted rule is to reinject cells at least 72 hours after the last dose of VP-16, although some authors postpone the reinfusion if plasma concentrations are above 0.3 µg/ml [28].

Drug Interactions

Phenytoin, anti-epileptic drugs and powerful hepatic enzyme inducers significantly increase the clearance of VP-16, i.e., reduce its plasma concentrations [26]. Phenytoin is often administered to prevent seizures caused by high-dose busulfan. It is well established that phenytoin also increases the clearance of busulfan. Thus, with all high-dose chemotherapy regimens necessitating seizure prophylaxis, benzodiazepines must be used and phenytoin and phenobarbital must be prohibited.

Toxicity of High-Dose VP-16

Toxicity During Administration of High-Dose VP-16

Approximately 50% of patients have nausea and vomiting, which is minimal to moderate and readily controlled by antiemetic drugs.
The reported frequency of fever, chills, episodes of hypotension and true anaphylactic reactions during VP-16 infusion varies from team to team. VP-16 solvents (polyethylene glycol, Tween-80 and ethanol) are often incriminated. The respective importance of the duration of infusion, VP-16 concentration and total dose is difficult to determine. Gianni reported that patients receiving methylprednisolone had no fever or chills, while 30% to 35% of those not receiving the steroid had these complications [10]. On the other hand, Chao reported that 40% of VP-16 infusions were associated with hypotension and hyperthermia despite

premedication with hydrocortisone and diphenhydramine [5]. Anaphylactic reactions (bronchospasm) are rare.
Between 10% and 40% of patients develop metabolic acidosis (fall in bicarbonates to as little as 10 mM), which is either asymptomatic or associated with hyperventilation. It is due to the PEG contained in the injectable form of VP-16. Some cases of confusion or disorientation during infusion of VP-16 have been attributed to the ethanol contained in the solution.

Haematological Toxicity

Haematological toxicity is not dose-limiting. Contrary to some alkylating agents, VP-16 spares multipotent bone marrow stem cells. It can be administered alone at high doses without the need for haematopoietic support.
In the study by Gianni, doses from 2 to 2.4 g/m^2 of VP-16 were administered as a single infusion lasting 10 to 12 h, with or without subsequent administration of a haematopoietic growth factor (G-CSF or GM-CSF) and without reinfusion of haematopoietic progenitor cells [10]. The median duration of neutropenia (< 500/mm^3) was 8 days without growth factors and 3 days with G-CSF or GM-CSF. Half the patients reached a platelet count of 100,000 after 13 days. Growth factors have no impact on the duration of thrombocytopenia. Platelet toxicity is weak, and is mainly observed in patients with bone marrow involvement.

Mucosal Toxicity

In dose escalation trials of VP-16 monotherapy, mucositis was virtually the only extra-haematopoietic form of toxicity. Its incidence and severity are linked to the total dose and probably to the duration of infusion, making it the dose-limiting toxic manifestation. The incidence and severity of mucosal lesions are increased when VP-16 is combined with TBI or alkylating agents such as busulfan and melphalan. With the conventional combination TBI-VP-16 (60 mg/kg in 3 to 5 hours), the incidence of severe mucositis necessitating major analgesics was 20% to 50%. Frequent mouthwashes during treatment can often attenuate mucositis.

Cutaneous Toxicity

A moderate skin rash can occur after VP-16 monotherapy. Postmus described the case of a patient who developed Stevens-Johnson syndrome after a dose of 2 g/m² [24]. The frequency of cutaneous toxicity is higher when VP-16 is administered in combination with other anticancer drugs. According to Giralt, 10% of patients receiving TBI + VP-16 + cyclophosphamide develop painful, desquamative erythrodermia of the palms and soles, associated with hypodermic oedema [11]. Bullous and desquamative erythrodermia is more frequent when VP-16 is combined with busulfan.

Other Forms of Toxicity

No renal, hepatic or pulmonary toxicity has been reported after high-dose VP-16 monotherapy. Hepatic toxicity, mainly in the form of veno-occlusive disease, is frequent when VP-16 is combined with busulfan, melphalan or TBI.

Antitumoural Activity

VP-16 is active against a wide variety of malignancies including blood cancers (leukaemia, lymphoma, Hodgkin's disease), malignant germ cell tumours, small-cell lung cancer and childhood malignancies [16]. VP-16 is used in several reference conditioning regimens, such as the VP-16 + cyclophosphamide + BCNU (CBV) combination for Hodgkin's disease [30], the VP-16 + BCNU + cytarabine + melphalan (BEAM) combination for non-Hodgkin's lymphomas [6], the TBI + VP-16 combination, with or without cyclophosphamide, before marrow allografting for acute leukaemia [2,4,11], and the VP-16 + cyclophosphamide + cisplatin or carboplatin (PEC and CarboPEC) combination for maligant germ cell tumours [17,25].

REFERENCES

1 Blume KG, Forman SJ, O'Donnell MR et al: Total body irradiation and high-dose etoposide: a new preparatory regimen for bone marrow transplantation in patients with advanced malignancies. Blood 1987 (69):1015-1020

2 Blume KG, Kopecky KJ, Henslee-Downey JP et al: A prospective randomized comparison of total body irradiation-etoposide versus busulfan-cyclophosphamide as preparatory regimens for bone marrow transplantation in patients with leukemia who were not in first remission: a Southwest Oncology Group study. Blood 1993 (81):2187-2193

3 Brown RA, Herzig RH, Wolff SN et al: High-dose etoposide and cyclophosphamide without bone marrow transplantation for resistant hematologic malignancy. Blood 1990 (76):473-479

4 Brown RA, Wolff SB, Fay JW et al: High-dose etoposide, cyclophosphamide, and total body irradiation with allogeneic bone marrow transplantation for patients with acute myeloid leukemia in untreated first relapse: a study by the North American Marrow Transplant group. Blood 1995 (85):1391-1395

5 Chao NJ, Stein AS, Long GD et al: Busulfan/etoposide: initial experience with a new preparatory regimen for autologous bone marrow transplantation in patients with acute non-lymphoblastic leukemia. Blood 1993 (81):319-323

6 Chopra R, McMillan AK, Linch DC et al: The place of high-dose BEAM therapy and autologous bone marrow transplantation in poor-risk Hodgkin's disease. A single-center eight-year study of 155 patients. Blood 1993 (81):1137-1145

7 Clark PI and Slevin ML: The clinical pharmacology of etoposide and teniposide. Clin Pharmacokinet 1987 (12):223-252

8 Creaven PJ: The clinical pharmacology of VM26 and VP16-213. Cancer Chemother Pharmacol 1982 (7):133-140

9 Creger RJ, Fox RM, Lazarus HM: Infusion of high doses of undiluted etoposide through central venous catheters during preparation for bone marrow transplantation. Cancer Invest 1990 (8):13-16

10 Gianni AM, Bregni M, Siena S et al: Granulocyte-macrophage colony-stimulating factor or granulocyte colony-stimulating factor infusion makes high-dose etoposide a safe outpatient regimen that is effective in lymphoma and myeloma patients. J Clin Oncol 1992 (10):1955-1962

11 Giralt SA, LeMaistre CF, Vriesendorp HM et al: Etoposide, cyclophosphamide, total-body irradiation, and allogeneic bone marrow transplantation for hematologic malignancies. J Clin Oncol 1994 (12):1923-1930

12 Gouyette A, Deniel A, Pico JL et al: Clinical pharmacology of high-dose etoposide associated with cisplatin: pharmacokinetic and metabolic studies. Eur J Clin Oncol 1987 (23):1623-1632

13 Greco FA, Johnson DH, Hainsworth JD: Chronic daily administration of oral etoposide. Semin Oncol 1990 (17 suppl 2):71-74

14 Hande KR, Wedlund PJ, Noone RM, Wilkinson GR, Greco FA, Wolff SN: Pharmacokinetics of high-dose

etoposide (VP-16-213) administered to cancer patients. Cancer Res 1984 (44):379-382

15 Henwood JM and Brogden RN: Etoposide: a review of its pharmacodynamic and pharmacokinetic properties, and therapeutic potential in combination chemotherapy of cancer. Drugs 1990 (39):438-490

16 Herzig RH: High-dose etoposide and marrow transplantation. Cancer 1991 (67):292-298

17 Ibrahim A, Zambon E, Bourhis JH et al: High-dose chemotherapy with etoposide, cyclophosphamide and escalating dose of carboplatin followed by autologous bone marrow transplantation in cancer patients. A pilot study. Eur J Cancer 1993 (29A):1398-1403

18 Joel SP, Clark PI, Maclean MC, Slevin ML: The stability of the intravenous preparation of etoposide in isotonic fluids. Proc Am Assoc Cancer Res 1989 (30):244 (abst)

19 Köhl P, Köppler H, Schmidt L, Fritsch HW, Holz J, Pflüger KH, Jungelas H: Pharmacokinetics of high-dose etoposide after short-term infusion. Cancer Chemother Pharmacol 1992 (29):316-320

20 Lazarus HM, Creger RJ, Diaz D: Simple method for the administration of high-dose etoposide during autologous bone marrow transplantation. Cancer Treat Rep 1984 (70):819-820

21 Lazarus HM, Gray R, Ciobanu N, Winter J, Weiner RS: Phase I trial of high-dose melphalan, high-dose etoposide and autologous bone marrow re-infusion in solid tumors: an Eastern Cooperative Oncology Group (ECOG) study. Bone Marrow Transplant 1994 (14):443-448

22 Mross K, Bewermeier P, Krüger W, Stockschläder M, Zander A, Hossfeld DK: Pharmacokinetics of undiluted or diluted high-dose etoposide with or without busulfan administered to patients with hematologic malignancies. J Clin Oncol 1994 (12):1468-1474

23 Mross KB: Safety, pharmacokinetics, and pharmacodynamics of high-dose etoposide (letter). J Clin Oncol 1994 (12):2768-2769

24 Postmus PE, Mulder NH, Sleijfer DT, Meinesz AF, Vriesendorp R, de Vries EGE: High-dose etoposide for refractory malignancies: a phase I study. Cancer Treat Rep 1984 (68):1471-1474

25 Pico JL, Droz JP, Ostronoff M: High-dose chemotherapy with autologous bone marrow transplantation for poor prognosis non-seminomatous germ cell tumors. In: Dicke KA, Spitzer G, Jagannath S et al (eds) Autologous Bone Marrow Transplantation: Proceedings of the Fourth International Symposium. Houston: University of Texas, MD Anderson Hospital and Tumor Institute, Scientific Publication 1989 pp 469-476

26 Rodman JH, Murry DJ, Madden T, Santana VM: Altered etoposide pharmacokinetics and time to engraftment in pediatric patients undergoing autologous bone marrow transplantation. J Clin Oncol 1994 (12):2390-2397

27 Schwinghammer TL: Safety, pharmacokinetics, and pharmacodynamics of high-dose etoposide (letter). J Clin Oncol 1994 (12):2768

28 Schwinghammer TL, Fleming RA, Rosenfeld CS, Przepiorka D, Shadduck RK, Bloom EJ, Stewart CF: Disposition of total and unbound etoposide followng high-dose therapy. Cancer Chemother Pharmacol 1993 (32):273-278

29 Stewart CF, Arbruck SG, Fleming RA, Evans WE: Changes in the clearance of total and unbound etoposide in patients with liver dysfunction. J Clin Oncol 1990 (8):1874-1879

30 Weaver CH, Appelbaum FR, Petersen FB et al: High-dose cyclophosphamide, carmustine, and etoposide followed by autologous bone marrow transplantation in patients with lymphoid malignancies who have received dose-limiting radiation therapy. J Clin Oncol 1993 (11):1329-1335

31 Wolff SN, Fer MF, McKay CM, Hande KR, Hainsworth JD, Greco FA: High-dose VP-16-213 and autologous bone marrow transplantation for refractory malignancies: a phase I study. J Clin Oncol 1983 (1):701-705

Intensive Sequential Chemotherapy for Untreated Poor-Risk Non-Hodgkin's Lymphoma

A.M. Stoppa, R. Bouabdallah, N. Vey, J.F. Rossi*, R. Costello, J. Camerlo,
G. Novakovitch, C. Chabannon, V.J. Bardou, D. Blaise, J.A. Gastaut and D. Maraninchi

Institut Paoli-Calmettes, 232 Boulevard Sainte Marguerite, 13273 Marseille
* Centre Hospitalier Regional Lapeyronie, 371 Avenue Doyen Giraud, 34295 Montpellier, France

First generation chemotherapy regimens like CHOP as well as second and third generation regimens - using multiple non-cross-resistant drugs and alternating cycles - have limited efficacy in high-risk non-Hodgkin's lymphomas (NHL). Recently, the age-adjusted International Prognostic Index (IPI) established for patients less than 60 years of age with intermediate or high grade histology that the presence of 2 or 3 risk factors leads to complete remission rates and 2-year survival inferior to 55%.

It is suspected that the limited activity of second and third generation regimens - even when adequately delivered with the support of granulocytic growth factors - is in part related to their moderate dose intensity increase when compared to standard CHOP. Major tolerable dose escalation has been achieved with several types of myeloablative regimens followed by autologous progenitor cell transplantation. These regimens are administered after previous induction chemotherapy and are mostly used as consolidation therapy in responding patients 3 to 6 months after diagnosis. This consolidation approach has resulted in up to 60% survival rates in selected patients.

Modern schedules for escalation of chemotherapy utilise growth factors and progenitor support to alter the established maximum tolerated dose, minimise the interval between cycles and maximise dose intensity, thus intensifying all aspects of treatment.

The use of such a strategy as front-line therapy rather than consolidation therapy may offer to more patients with aggressive lymphoma the potential benefits of dose size and dose intensity of the most active drugs.

Conventional Chemotherapy

In the last two decades, numerous combinations of chemotherapy regimens have been devised for the treatment of aggressive NHL in intermediate or high grade histology patients. First generation CHOP-like regimens established that administration of doxorubicin, cyclophosphamide, vincristine and prednisone for 6 to 8 cycles given every 3 weeks, can cure 30% of these patients.

Second and third generation regimens reinforced the CHOP frame with additional drugs (methotrexate, bleomycin, etoposide) given as successive or alternating cycles (CAPBOP, mBACOD, MACOPB, PROMACE MOPP, PROMACE CYTABOM) in order to counteract the naturally developing resistance of aggressive lymphoma by multiple drug administration and increased doses [1-5]. The last generation regimens have the same objective and consist of sequential regimens with successive, different drug cocktails (Vanderbilt, LNH80, 84, 87; CHOP/VIMB) [6-8] (Table 1).

Despite encouraging early results, it does not seem that second and third generation regimens offer any advantage in outcome over CHOP. When CHOP, mBACOD, MACOPB and PROMACE CYTABOM were compared in a controlled study, no differences were observed in complete remission (CR), overall survival (OS) and disease-free survival (DFS) rates, which were 50%, 48% and 43%, respectively [1]. The experience accumulated over the years with the treatment of aggressive lymphoma has, however, put into evi-

Table 1. Conventional chemotherapy

Author	Regimen	No. pts.	Selection	CR	O S	DFS	FFS
Fisher*	CHOP or mBACOP or Promace Cytabom or MACOPB	899	II bulky III - IV	44% 48% 56% 51%	54% (3y) 52% (3y) 50% (3y) 50% (3y)	41% 46% 46% 41%	-
Zuckerman	AVPAC AVAD EVDAC	150	II - III - IV	83% 72% 76%	-		62% (5y) 51% (5y) 59% (5y)
Somers*	Promace MOPP or CHVMP - VP	346	II bulky III - IV	48% 61%	52% IPI / PR = 30% (5y)	60%	48%
Vose	CAPBOP regimen CBA CBA1 CBM	389	II bulky III - IV	 69% 73% 71%	 50% 56% 47% IPI / PR 33-45% (3y)		IPI / PR 20%
MacMaster	Vanderbilt regimen	56	expected cure <25%	77%	-	-	52% (5y)
Sertoli*	MACOPB or Promace MOPP	221	bulky	50%	50% (3y)	-	36%
Delena	CEOP VIMB	60	III - IV	77%	77% (4y) IPI / PR 0-65%	83% IPI / PR 0-50%	-

* : randomised study   IPI / PR : International Prognostic Index / poor risk = 2 or 3 risk factors   y : year

dence three major points which form a basis of reflection for modern strategies.

Risk Factors

Univariate analysis recognises 10 risk factors (RF) associated with the achievement of CR and long-term survival (age, performance status, B symptoms, Ann Arbor stage, mass size, number of extranodal sites, bone marrow involvement, serum LDH, serum β_2-microglobulin, serum albumin). In 1993 the International Non-Hodgkin's Lymphoma Prognostic Factor Project established 5 risk factors (age >60, extranodal tumours ≥2, stage ≥III, LDH >normal value, ECOG performance status ≥2), the presence of which identified 4 risk groups. This index has been adjusted for patients below the age of 60. In 1274 patients (60 years old or younger) tumour stage, LDH and ECOG identified 4 risk groups with predicted 5-year survival rates of 83%, 69%, 46%, 32% depending on the presence of 0, 1, 2 or 3 risk factors [9].

The Importance of Achieving CR

The definition of CR is not yet uniform. Apart from the disappearance of all lesions, the significance of residual masses, particularly in patients with bulky tumours, can be difficult to decide upon. Despite the heterogeneity of definitions, not achieving CR is still the worst prognostic factor for outcome. Patients with resistant disease die rapidly and patients with partial responses (defined as an at least 50% reduction of all tumour lesions) have a 2-year survival below 30% compared to 80-100% for patients achieving CR [10].

Role of Dose Intensity

Retrospective studies of the actual relative dose intensity (received dose/planned dose) revealed that the relative dose intensity (DI) of cyclophosphamide and doxorubicin is predictive of response and survival, with a worse outcome for patients receiving less than 75% of the planned dose [11-15]. The failure of second and third regimens to improve outcome might be related to the fact that, as drugs are not equally active, in most cases the addition of new drugs requires decreased doses of the most active agents of the gold standard (cyclophosphamide, anthracycline) to avoid unacceptable toxicity.

Dose Escalation and Place of Growth Factors

Although it has been established that decreased DI negatively affects the outcome of patients with aggressive NHL, no randomised study has yet determined whether the same combination regimen used at an increased DI is associated with an improved survival rate.

The use of granulocytic growth factors (GF) G-CSF or GM-CSF after conventionally dosed regimens has made it possible to respect the planned dose and schedule of chemotherapy. However, this did not result in improved CR and survival rates, probably because the differences in DI of the GF-supported or non-supported groups were small [16-19]. Thus it is generally assumed that the impact of DI escalation will be minimal. This assumption might change if the DI increase is substantial.

Pilot studies have shown that addition of G-CSF or GM-CSF allows patients to tolerate a 2-fold increase in the cyclophosphamide dose of standard CHOP over 6 cycles and, in one study, a 2-fold increase in the 4 EPI adriamycin dose as well [20-22].

Two phase I studies have been conducted using G-CSF or GM-CSF to increase the maximum tolerated doses of the PROMACE CYTABOM and CHOP regimens. In the first study, cyclophosphamide (day 1), doxorubicin (day 1), etoposide (day 1), and cytarabine (day 8) were escalated up to 200% of the standard combination dose for 6 cycles at 21-day intervals, GM-CSF being administered from day 9 to 19. Median grade 4 neutropenia lasted 1.5 day at the 200% dose level, which was defined as the maximum tolerated dose (MTD), but no grade 4 thrombocytopenia occurred. The authors pointed out that the dose intensity achieved for the day-8 drugs was lower than that of the day-1 drugs and that DI decreased over time with the repetition of the

cycles due to delayed haematological recovery [23].

In the second study, cyclophosphamide and doxorubicin were escalated up to 530% and 140% (MTD), respectively, of the standard CHOP doses for a total of 4 cycles administered every 3 weeks with the support of G-CSF. At the MTD, 65% of the cycles were complicated by febrile neutropenia and 84% of patients received at least one platelet transfusion. The median duration of grade 4 thrombopenia ($<20 \times 10^9$/L) increased with the repetition of the cycles. Stem cell toxicity was suggested by the fact that after the fourth and last cycle the median time to recover 90 $\times 10^9$/L platelets was 29 days, with 26% of the patients requiring 7 weeks.

This study reported an encouraging CR rate (86%) with an OS of 70% at 2 years for the 22 poor risk patients treated at the MTD level [24].

These two studies suggest that substantial dose intensity can be obtained with the support of growth factors but probably not over a prolonged period of time, thrombocytopenia being the new dose limiting toxicity. Thus the total administered doses might be less than expected.

For example, the highest DI currently obtained with the high-dose CHOP regimen (cyclophosphamide 530%, doxorubicin 140% of standard CHOP) does not result in the same increase in the cumulative doses (cyclophosphamide 350%, doxorubicin 93% of standard CHOP) because of the different duration of therapy (12 weeks vs 18 weeks) (see Table 4).

Role of High-Dose Therapy and Progenitor Cell Rescue

Considering the difficulty to maintain high dose intensity over more than 3 months, an alternative way to achieve substantial cumulative doses of active drugs is to deliver high doses of alkylating agents (cyclophosphamide, melphalan, BCNU, total body irradiation) supported by autologous bone marrow (BM) or peripheral blood progenitor cells (PBPC), which ensure full haematological recovery. The limiting toxicity of these conditioning regimens (BEAM, BEAC, CBV, Cy TBI) is associated with non-haematological toxicity, mainly diges-

Table 2. High-dose therapy with autologous bone marrow transplantation

Author	Regimen	No. pts.	Status	Selection	CR	OS	DFS	FFS
Sweetenham	Chemo TBI/ABMT	102	CR1	II bulky III - IV	-	70% (4y)	70%	-
Vittolo	MACOPB + MitoARAC + BEAM/ABMT	57	untreated	DLC bulky II - III - IV	76%	-	77% (2y)	-
Milpied	Sequential chemo + BEAM/ABMT	102	untreated	bulky II - III - IV	-	60% (3y)	-	55%
Gherlinzoni *	DHAP or CBV/ABMT	51	PR1	PR1	55% 95%	58% 81%** (3y)	49% 72%**	
Verdonck*	CHOP x 4 or CyTBI/ABMT	69	PR1	PR1	74% 68%	85% 56% (2y)	72% 60%	53% 41%
Haioun*	LNH87 chemo or CBV/ABMT	64	PR1	PR1 IPI / PR	-	46% 63%** (5y)	-	20% 58%**
Haioun*	LNH87 chemo or CBV/ABMT	236	CR1	IPI / PR	-	52% 63%** (5y)	36% 57%**	-
Gianni*	MACOPB or intensive chemo + CyTBI/ABMT	75	untreated	bulky II - III - IV	61% 94%**	-	-	40% 75%** (3y)

* : randomised study   ** : $p < 0.05$ IPI / PR : International Prognostic Index / poor risk = 2 or 3 risk factors
DLC : diffuse large cells

tive toxicity. The procedure, which is still restricted to patients below 60 years of age, is now safe, with a mortality rate reduced to 1-5% in chemosensitive patients.

Over the last 5 years, high-dose therapy has become the standard for certain categories of patients (Table 2).

The Parma study has established the benefit of the BEAC regimen followed by autologous peripheral cell transplantation (APCT) in the treatment of sensitive relapses, with 50% of patients being cured versus 30% of those receiving the DHAP chemotherapy regimen [25].

The value of salvage of partial remissions with APCT is still not clear: two studies report an advantage of APCT over consolidation with the LNH87 or DHAP regimens and one study reports identical results with APCT or prolonged CHOP therapy [26-28].

Uncontrolled pilot studies involving poor-risk patients (generally bulky disease or Ann Arbor stage IV) in CR1 or very good first partial remission (VGPR1) have shown that APCT helps to obtain long-term survival in 70% of patients in CR1 or VGPR1 [29,30].

Recently the GELA group, in the LNH87 study, reported improved overall survival and disease-free survival for patients with 2 or 3 risk factors who received CBV followed by APCT in CR1 as compared to a conventional consolidation arm (5-year DFS 57% versus 36%) [31].

High-Dose Therapy - Open Questions

Patient Selection

At present the impact of high-dose therapy is established mostly in chemosensitive patients. In the LNH87 study, where the advantage of intensification has been clearly demonstrated, 30% of the patients in the high and high/intermediate risk category were not eligible for randomisation. Thus failure-free survival (based on patient observation from the time of diagnosis) gives the best estimation of cure. This evaluation has not been regularly reported in high-dose therapy studies. The Goelam group reported the outcome of 162 untreated poor-risk patients submitted to conventional dose reduction therapy and BEAM/APCT with a 3-year failure-free survival of 50% [32].

Gianni reported on an original and encouraging approach of sequential, time and dose-intensive single agent administration followed by Melphalan TBI/APCT. The report showed a CR and FFS advantage compared to a historical series of poor-risk patients treated with MACOBB [33].

Progenitor Cell Contamination

During the past 5 years, progenitor cell collection from peripheral blood (PBPC) by apheresis after priming by G-CSF or GM-CSF, or at the leukocyte rebound following chemotherapy, has progressively supplanted bone marrow (BM) harvest. Apart from the uniform patient preference for this procedure and the logistic advantage, faster platelet recovery and shorter hospitalisation have been established in a randomised study [34].

Tumour cell contamination of progenitor cell infusion has been reported to alter the outcome following APCT, especially in low grade follicular lymphoma [35]. It is commonly assumed that PBPC might be less contaminated than BM harvest. Sharp recently reported that lymphoma cells, identified by clonogenic assay or clonal T cell, IgH rearrangement, were present in the apheresis product in only 2/20 patients with histologically involved bone marrow. The outcome after APCT for these 20 patients was comparable to that of 45 patients transplanted with autologous non-involved bone marrow [36].

Secondary Leukaemia

There is concern about a significant cumulative incidence of myelodysplasia (MDS) or secondary acute myeloid leukaemia following high-dose alkylating agents. The EBMT registry reported in 2354 lymphoma patients receiving APCT a 4% incidence at 5 years with 14%, 6% and 0.4% for low-grade lymphoma, Hodgkin's lymphoma and non-low-grade NHL, respectively. The lower frequency in the latter group adds weight to the hypothesis that post-transplantation MDS reflects the effects of prior chemotherapy rather than toxicity from the procedure itself [37].

Cost

The use of peripheral blood progenitor cells instead of bone marrow should result in cost savings of approximately 30% per transplant. Nevertheless, dose intensification with progenitor cell support after CBV, BEAM or CyTBI regimens will require hospitalisation for a median of 3 weeks in a transplant unit. The cost and availability of such units can be prohibitive.

Intensive Sequential Chemotherapy with Repeated Growth Factor and Progenitor Cell Support

The concept that a high dose intensity and a high total dose delivered should have a positive impact on CR and FFS, along with the availability of GFs and progenitor cells, has led to the development of modern regimens supported by repeated GF and progenitor cell administration in order to improve cure rates.

Most of the studies conducted so far have dealt with carboplatin, cyclophosphamide and etoposide combinations in solid tumours and have shown that PBPC and GF support reduce the myelotoxicity, thus improving chemotherapy delivery and allowing regularly tolerated doses of up to 200% of the standard regimen [38-41].

Wheeler followed the same approach in refractory or relapsed Hodgkin's and non-Hodgkin's lymphoma. Patients were submitted to repeated high-dose ICE with progenitor cell support followed by CBV/APCT. In this study 70% of patients had objective responses and could undergo CBV/APCT.

Marseille Experience with Poor-Risk Non-Hodgkin's Lymphoma

We have explored this strategy in two consecutive trials (ISC92 and ISC95) in which intensive sequential chemotherapy regimens were given as first-line therapy to high and high/intermediate risk NHL patients, with the aim of measuring the efficacy of PBPC to support full dose administration in an outpatient setting. Thirty-five patients with aggressive histology and poor risk factors according to age-adjusted IPI entered ISC92 (n=20) and ISC95 (n=15) from October 1992 to September 1995. The median age was 41 years (range 20-60), 24/35 were in the high/intermediate (2 risk factors) and 11/35 in the high (3 risk factors) risk categories (Table 3).

ISC92 (October 1992 - March 1995) delivered 6 cycles at 3-week intervals including 3 induction cycles (A1, A2, A3 Cy 3000 mg/m^2, Doxo 75 mg/m^2) followed by 3 intensified progenitor cell supported cycles (B4, B5, B6 Cy 3000 mg/m^2, Doxo 75 mg/m^2, VP-16 300 mg/m^2, CDDP 100 mg/m^2) (Table 3, Fig. 1).

Table 3. ISC92-95 regimens

ISC92		ISC95	
A1-A2-A3		**A1**	
Cy	3000 mg/m^2 d1	Cy	500 mg/m^2 d1
Doxo	75 mg/m^2 d1	VCR	2 mg/m^2 d1
VCR	2 mg/m^2 d1	Prednisone d 1-5	
Prednisone d 1-5			
		A2	
		Cy	6000 mg/m^2 d1
		Doxo	75 mg/m^2 d1
		VCR	2 mg/m^2 d1
		Prednisone d 1-5	
		A3	
		Cy	4000 mg/m^2 d1
		Doxo	75 mg/m^2 d1
		VCR	2 mg/m^2 d1
		Prednisone d 1-5	
B4-B5-B6		**B4-B5**	
Cy	3000 mg/m^2 d1	Cy	4000 mg/m^2 d1
Doxo	75 mg/m^2 d1	Doxo	75 mg/m^2 d1
VCR	2 mg/m^2 d1	VCR	2 mg/m^2 d1
VP-16	300 mg/m^2 d2	VP-16	500 mg/m^2 d2
CDDP	100 mg/m^2 d2	CDDP	100 mg/m^2 d2
Prednisone d 1-5		ARAC	1000 mg/m^2 d2
		Prednisone d 1-5	

d : day   Cy : cyclophosphamide   Doxo : doxorubicin   VCR : vincristine   VP-16 : etoposide   CDDP : cisplatin
ARAC : cytarabine

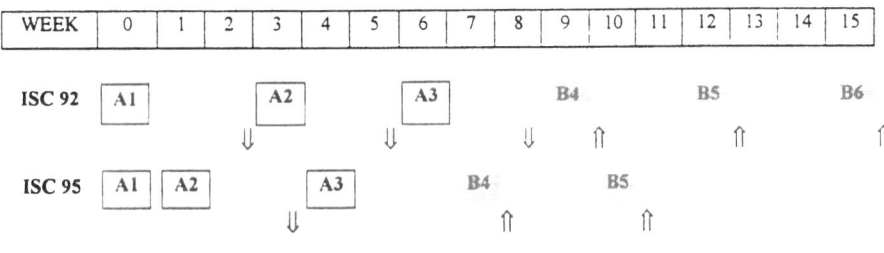

WEEK	0	1	2	3	4	5	6	7	8	9	10	11	12	13	14	15

Fig 1. ISC92 and 95 regimens   ⇓ Apheresis
                                         ⇑ infusion

ISC95 (start April 1995) began with low-dose CHOP (A1) followed by 4 cycles delivered at 3-week intervals including 2 induction cycles (A2 = Cy 6000 mg/m², Doxo 75 mg/m², A3 = Cy 4000 mg/m², Doxo 75 mg/m²) and 2 intensified progenitor cell supported cycles B4, B5 (Cy 4000 mg/m², Doxo 75 mg/m², VP-16 500 mg/ m², CDDP 100 mg/m², Arac 1000 mg/m²) (Fig. 1).

The duration of therapy [(day 1 last cycle - day 1 first cycle) + 3 weeks] was 18 and 13 weeks for ISC92 and ISC95, respectively. Condition of administration of chemotherapy required 1 x 10⁹/L polymorphonuclear cells and 90 x 10⁹/L platelets.

Filgrastim and oral antibioprophylaxis were given after each cycle from day 6 up to neutrophil reconstitution (1 x 10⁹/L).

Apheresis was performed after the A cycles and its product was reinfused after each B cycle to ensure adequate haematopoietic recovery for subsequent chemotherapy administration.

The total median number of CD34-positive cells per kg body weight collected was 16 x 10⁶ (3.3-30). A minimum of 2 x 10⁶/kg CD34 cells were always available for each intensified B cycle except in one patient. Lymphoma cells were not detected by cytological analysis.

Haematological toxicity increased with the repetition of the cycles. Median grade 4 neutropenia (0.5 x 10⁹/L) was 2 days (0-9) and 4 days (1-10) for A and B cycles, respectively (p = 0.09). Readmission for febrile neutropenia was more frequent (p= 0.05) during B cycles (60%) than during A cycles (38%). The median duration of each hospital stay was 6 days (4-21). The median duration of grade 4 thrombocytopenia (<20 x 10⁹/L) was longer (p < 0.001) during B cycles [6 days (1-21)] than during A cycles [0 days (0-4)]. All patients received at

least one platelet transfusion. Platelet requirement was more frequent (p < 0.01) during B cycles (63%) than during A cycles (9%).

Chemotherapy delivery was satisfactory. The 35 patients received 174 cycles of the 180 cycles planned. All the A cycles (90/90) were administered and 91% of them were delayed less than 3 days. Ninety-four per cent (84/90) of the B cycles were administered and 71% of them were delayed less than 3 days.

The median actual relative dose intensity (actual received dose/planned dose) for cyclophosphamide and doxorubicin was 94% (50-100). Eighty per cent of the patients received more than 75% of the planned dose. Cumulative dose, dose intensity and comparison with standard CHOP or different regimens are listed in Table 4.

After the last cycle the overall response rate was 85% including 24/35 complete responses (68%) and 6/35 partial responses (17%). One patient died of pneumopathy and 4 were refractory. With a median follow-up of 18 months (range 9-45 months), 9 relapses occurred (5/6 PR-4/24 CR) within a median of 6 months (range 3-20).

The projected 2-year survival, disease-free survival and failure-free survival are 75%, 72% and 52%, respectively.

A cost analysis was performed on the first 20 patients in the ISC92 trial (Table 5). It included the cost of chemotherapy (drugs, filgrastim, transfusion), progenitor cells (collection, cryopreservation, infusion), hospitalisation for chemotherapy administration, febrile neutropenia and systematic consultation twice a week. The total cost of the procedure was superposable to the cost of the intensified BEAM regimen with PBPC in the same institution (19750 versus 19770 US dollars). Thus we may probably assume that treatment with intensive se-

Table 4a. Dose intensity and comparison with standard CHOP

Regimen	Duration (weeks)	Cyclophosphamide mg/m²/week	Doxorubicin mg/m²/week
CHOP	18	250 (1)	16.6 (1)
mBACOD	18	200 (0.8)	15 (0.89)
MACOPB	18	175 (0.7)	25 (1.5)
Promace Cytabom Standard	18	217 (0.86)	8 (0.5)
Promace Cytabom MTD*	18	417 (1.66)	15 (0.9)
Vanderbilt	9	500 (2)	10 (0.2)
ACVBP (LNH87)	9	533 (2.1)	333 (2)
CHOP* MTD	12	1333 (5.3)	23 (1.4)
ISC92**	18	1000 (4)	25 (1.5)
ISC95**	13	1423 (5.6)	23 (1.4)

* : supported by G-CSF or GM-CSF   ** : supported by G-CSF and progenitor cells
( ) : dose intensity / dose intensity standard CHOP
NB duration of therapy = (day 1 last cycle - day 1 first cycle) + 3 weeks

Table 4b. Cumulative doses and comparison with standard CHOP

Regimen	Duration (weeks)	Cyclophosphamide mg/m²	Doxorubicin mg/m²	VP-16	ARAC
CHOP	18	4500 (1)	300 (1)		
mBACOD	18	3800 (0.8)	270 (0.9)		
MACOPB	18	3150 (0.7)	450 (1.5)		
Promace Cytabom Standard	18	3900 (0.86)	150 (0.5)	960	1800
Promace Cytabom MTD*	18	7800 (1.73)	300 (1)	1920	3600
Vanderbilt	9	4500 (1)	90 (0.3)	1500	
LNH 87 ACVBP* + consolidation	16	6300 (1.4)	300 (1)	600	800
CHOP MTD*	12	16000 (3.5)	280 (0.9)		
ISC92**	18	18000 (4)	450 (1.5)	900	
ISC95**	13	18500 (4.1)	300 (1)	1000	2000

* : supported by G-CSF or GM-CSF   ** : supported by G-CSF and progenitor cells
( ) : total dose / total dose standard CHOP
NB duration of therapy = (day 1 last cycle - days 1 first cycle) + 3 weeks

Table 5. ISC92 cost analysis

Chemotherapy		3961
	drugs	1197
	filgrastim	710
	transfusions	2054
Progenitor cells		2346
	collection, cryopreservation, infusion	
Hospitalisation		13434
	chemotherapy	1728
	febrile neutropenia	4420
	consultation	7296
Total	US $	19750

quential chemotherapy is less expensive than conventional chemotherapy regimen induction, i.e. CHOP for 4 courses, followed by BEAM intensification [43].

From these two consecutive studies we conclude that repeated GF and progenitor cell support allow delivery on an outpatient basis of a very high dose intensity regimen (400% to 500% increased Cy dose of standard CHOP, 140% to 150% increased Doxo dose of standard CHOP) for a prolonged period of time (13 to 18 weeks).

Although not randomised, our studies showed encouraging CR (68%) and 2-year survival (75%) rates when compared to conventional chemotherapy studies which classically report CR and survival of less than 55% in similar categories of patients (Fig. 2).

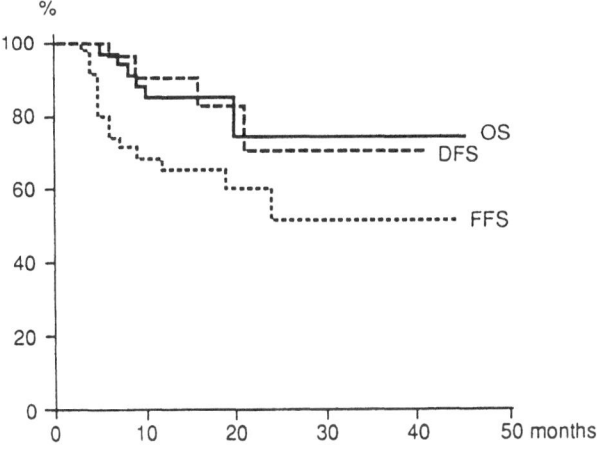

Fig. 2. ISC92-95 outcome

Prospects

The relevance of upfront high-dose chemotherapy in NHL is based on evidence accumulated over the years showing that poor-risk NHL patients could benefit from a major increase in dose intensity and/or dose size of the most active drugs.

At the present time, trials are conducted comparing the impact of one versus two intensification chemotherapy regimens (LNH93) as well as a large scale phase II study of high-dose CHOP in this subset of patients with the expectation that higher doses will lead to higher CR and FFS rates.

Peripheral blood progenitor cell supported therapy represents a technological breakthrough:

1. Systematic support with GF and PBPC of very high-dose chemotherapy can be safely administered in an outpatient setting outside the transplant unit.
2. Concern about tumour cell contamination will decrease by improving residual disease detection (clonal IgH, TcR) and progenitor cell purification.
3. If upfront, very high-dose intensity regimens can be of benefit to unselected poor-risk NHL patients, intensive sequential chemotherapy with progenitor cell support allowing the optimisation of drug delivery should improve the overall cure rate in this disease. Larger cohorts of patients are needed to validate the possibility of diffusion of the procedure in small centres.
4. As clinical conditioning regimens followed by PBPC have become the standard therapy used by increasing numbers of oncological teams, randomised studies will ultimately be required.

REFERENCES

1   Fisher RI, Gaynor ER, Dahlberg S et al: Comparison of a standard regimen (CHOP) with three intensive chemotherapy regimens for advanced non-Hodgkin's lymphoma. N Engl J Med 1993 (328): 1002-1006

2   Zuckerman KS: Efficacy of intensive, high-dose anthracycline-based therapy in intermediate and high-grade non Hodgkin's lymphomas. Sem Oncol 1994 (21 Suppl 1):59-64

3   Somers R, Carde P, Thomas J et al: EORTC study of non Hodgkin's lymphoma: Phase III study comparing CHVmP-VB and ProMACE-MOPP in patients with stage II, III and IV intermediate and high grade lymphoma. Ann Oncol 1994 (5 Suppl 2):S85-S89

4   Vose JM, Anderson JR, Bierman PJ et al: Comparison of front line chemotherapy for aggressive non Hodgkin lymphoma using the CAP-BOP regimens. Sem Hematol 1994 (31 Suppl 3):4-8

5   Sertoli MR, Santini G, Chisesi T et al: MACOP-B versus ProMACE-MOPP in the treatment of advanced diffuse non-Hodgkin's lymphoma: Results of a prospective randomized trial by the non-Hodgkin's lymphoma cooperative study group. J Clin Oncol 1994 (12):1366-1374

6   McMaster ML, Greer JP, Wolff SN et al: Results of treatment with high intensity brief duration chemotherapy in poor prognosis non-Hodgkin's lymphoma. Cancer 1991 (2):233-241

7   De Lena M, Ditonno P, Lorusso V et al: CEOP-B alternated with VIMB in intermediate grade and high grade non Hodgkin's lymphoma: A pilot study. J Clin Oncol 1995 (13):953-960

8   Haioun C, Lepage E, Gisselbrecht et al: Comparison of autologous bone marrow transplantation with sequential chemotherapy for intermediate grade and high grade non-Hodgkin's lymphoma in first complete remission: A study of 464 patients. J Clin Oncol 1994 (12):2543-2551

9   Shipp S et al: A predictive model for aggressive non Hodgkin's lymphoma. The International non-Hodgkin's lymphoma prognostic factors project. N Engl J Med 1993 (329):987-997

10   Hacq R, Sawka CA, Franssen E et al: Significance of a partial or slow response to front line chemotherapy in the management of intermediate grade or high grade non-Hodgkin's lymphoma: A literature review. J Clin Oncol 1994 (12):1074-1084

11   Hrymink WM and Goodyear M: The calculation of received dose intensity. J Clin Oncol 1990 (8):1935-1937

12   Kwak LW, Halpern J, Olshen A et al: Prognostic significance of actual dose intensity in diffuse large cell lymphoma: Results of a tree-structured survival analysis. J Clin Oncol (8):963-977

13   Epelbaum R, Faraggi D, Ben-Arie Y et al: Survival of diffuse large cell lymphoma. Cancer 1990 (66):1124-1129

14   Meyer RM, Hryniuk WM, Goodyear DE: The role of dose intensity in determining outcome in intermediate grade non-Hodgkin's lymphoma. J Clin Oncol 1991 (9):339-341

15   Lepage E, Gisselbrecht C, Haioun C et al: Prognostic significance of received relative dose intensitu in non-Hodgkin's lymphoma patients: Application to LNH-87 protocol. Ann Oncol 1993 (4):651-656

16   Pettengell R, Gurney H, Radford JA et al: Granulocyte colony stimulating factor to prevent dose-limiting neutropenia in non-Hodgkin's lymphoma: a randomized controlled trial. Blood 1992 (80):1430-1436

17   Gerhartz HH, Engelhard M, Meusers P et al: Randomized, double blind, placebo controlled phase III study of recombinant human granulocyte macrophage colony-stimulating factor as adjunct to induction treatment of high-grade malignant non-Hodgkin's lymphomas. Blood 1993 (82):2329-2339

18   Avilés A, Diaz-Maqueo JC, Talavera A et al: Effect of granulocyte colony stimulating factor in patients with diffuse large cell lymphoma treated with intensive chemotherapy. Leukemia and Lymphoma 1994 (15):153-157

19   Engelhard M, Gerhartz H, Brittinger G et al: Cytokine efficiency in the treatment of high-grade malignant non-Hodgkin's lymphomas: Results of a randomized double blind placebo controlled study with intensified COP-BLAM ± rhGM-CSF. Ann Oncol 1994 (5 Suppl 1):S213

20   Grigg A, Wolf M, Levi J et al: Escalated dose epirubicin cyclophosphamide with filgrastim for patients with aggressive non-Hodgkin's lymphoma. Proc ASCO 1995 (12) 1255:411

21   Shambaugh S, Belman N, Ehmann WC et al: Dose-intensified chemotherapy for intermediate grade non-Hodgkin lymphoma. Proc ASCO 1995 (12) 1296a:421

22   Casanova L, Gomez H, Kahatt C et al: Biweekly intensified CHOP (I-CHOP) regimen using GM-CSF 5MOLGRAMOSTIM) in aggressive non Hodgkin's lymphoma. Proc ASCO 1995 (12) 1303a:423

23   Gordon LI, Andersen J, Habermann TM et al: Phase I trial of dose escalation with growth factor support in patients with previously untreated diffuse aggressive lymphomas: determination of the maximum tolerated dose of ProMACE-CytaBOM. J Clin Oncol 1996 (14):1275-1281

24   Shipp MA, Neuberg D, Janicek M et al: High dose CHOP as initial therapy for patients with poor prognosis aggressive non-Hodgkin's lymphoma: a dose-finding pilot study. J Clin Oncol 1995 (13):2916-2923

25   Philip T, CGuglielmi C, Hagenbeek A et al: Autologous bone marrow transplantation as compared with salvage chemotherapy in relapses of chemotherapy sensitive non-Hodgkin's lymphoma. N Engl J Med 1995 (333):1540-1545

26   Haioun C, Lepage E, Gisselbrecht E et al: Autologous bone marrow transplantation versus sequential chemotherapy for aggressive non-Hodgkin's lymphoma partially responding to first line chemotherapy: A study of 96 patients enrolled in the LNH87 protocol. Blood 1995 (86 Suppl 1):a823

27   Gherlinzoni F, Martelli M, Mazza P et al: Autologous bone marrow transplantation versus DHAP in aggressive non-Hodgkin's lymphomas partially responding to first line chemotherapy. Blood 1994 (84):a234 (abstr 922)

28 Verdonck LF, Van Putten WLJ, Hagenbeek A et al: Comparison of CHOP chemotherapy with autologous bone marrow transplantation for slowly responding patients with aggressive non-Hodgkin's lymphoma. N Engl J Med 1995 (332):1045-1051

29 Sweetenham JW, Proctor SJ, Blaise D et al: High dose therapy and autologous bone marrow transplantation in first complete remission for adult patients with high-grade non-Hodgkin's lymphoma: The EBMT experience. Ann Oncol 1994 (5 Suppl 2): S155-S159

30 Vitolo U, Cortellazzo S, Liberati AM et al: Intensified chemotherapy followed by myeloablative therapy and autologous stem cell transplantation as first line therapy in high risk diffuse large cell lymphoma. Blood 1995 (86 Suppl 1) a1819:458

31 Haioun C, Lepage E, Gisselbrecht C et al: Autologous bone marrow transplantation versus sequential chemotherapy for aggressive non-Hodgkin's lymphoma in first complete remission: A study of 542 patients (LNH-87 protocol). Blood 1995 (86 Suppl 1):a1816

32 Milpied N, Lamy T, Gaillard F et al: Intensive short term therapy for adults with disseminated intermediate or high grade non Hodgkin's lymphomas: Analysis of prognostic factors in a prospective multicenter trial. BMT 1990 (17 Suppl 1):S30

33 Gianni AM, Bregni M, Siena S et al: Five-year update of the Milan Cancer Institute randomized trial of high-dose sequential versus MACOP-B therapy for diffuse large-cell lymphomas. Proc Annual Meeting ASCO 1994 (13):A1263

34 Schmitz N, Linch DC, Dreger P et al: Randomised trial of filgrastim mobilised peripheral blood progenitor cell transplantation versus autologous bone marrow transplantation in lymphoma patients. The Lancet 1996 (347):353-357

35 Gribben JG, Freedmon AS, Neuberg D et al: Immunologic purging of marrow assessed by PCR before autologous bone marrow transplantation for B-cell lymphoma. N Engl J Med 1991 (325):1525-1533

36 Sharp JG, Kessinger A, Mann S et al: Outcome of high-dose therapy and autologous transplantation in non-Hodgkin's lymphoma based on the presence of tumor in the marrow or infused hematopoietic harvest. J Clin Oncol1996 (14):214-219

37 Milligan DW, Kolb HJ, Pearce R et al: MDS after autografting for lymphoma: A retrospective analysis of the EBMT registry. BMT 1996 (17 Suppl 1):a634

38 Shea TC, Mason JR, Storniolo AM et al: Sequential cycles of high-dose carboplatin administered with recombinant human granulocyte macrophage colony stimulating factor and repeated infusions of autologous peripheral blood progenitor cells: A novel and effective method for delivering multiple courses of dose intensive therapy. J Clin Oncol 1992 (10):464-473

39 Tepler I, Cannistra SA, Frei E et al: Use of peripheral blood progenitor cells abrogates the myelotoxicity of repetitive outpatient high-dose carboplatin and cyclophosphamide chemotherapy. J Clin Oncol 1993 (11):1583-1591

40 Fennelly D, Wasserheit C, Schneider J et al: Simultaneous dose escalating and schedule intensification of carboplatin based chemotherapy using peripheral blood progenitor cells and filgrastim: A phase I trial. Cancer Res 1994 (54):6137-6142

41 Pettengell R, Woll PJ, Tatcher N et al: Multicyclic, dose-intensive chemotherapy supported by sequential reinfusion of hematopoietic progenitors in whole blood. J Clin Oncol 1995 (13):148-156

42 Wheeler C, Shulman LN, Elias A et al: Sequential ifosfamide, carboplatin and etoposide with steroids and cyclophosphamide (Cy/AG-CSF) mobilized peripheral blood progenitor cell (PBPC) support (SPICE) in relapsed lymphomas. Proc Am Soc Clin Oncol 1995 (14):913A

43 Faucher C, Le Corroller AG, Blaise D et al: Comparison of G-CSF primed peripheral blood progenitor cells and bone marrow autotransplantation: Clinical assessment and cost-effectiveness. BMT 1994 (14):895-901

High-Dose Chemotherapy with Autologous Haematopoietic Progenitor Cell Transplantation for Adenocarcinoma of the Breast

Jared L. Klein and William P. Peters

Barbara Ann Karmanos Cancer Institute, Wayne State University School of Medicine, Detroit, Michigan 48201, U.S.A.

Breast cancer is the second most common malignancy of women in the United States. One hundred and eighty-five thousand new cases are estimated to occur each year and approximately 44,300 women will die this year from breast cancer. No curable regimen including conventional-dose chemotherapy or hormonal therapy has been found for metastatic breast cancer. Although 10-35% of patients will achieve a complete remission with conventional-dose chemotherapy, the median duration of survival is approximately 1-2 years for patients with metastatic breast cancer [1]. These frustrating results prompted the exploration of high-dose chemotherapy for breast cancer and it is now more than a decade since the initial efforts to use high-dose chemotherapy with autologous bone marrow transplantation for patients with metastatic breast cancer. Over this time, the use of this treatment approach has massively expanded and breast cancer is now the most common disease in which high-dose chemotherapy and autologous haematopoietic progenitor cell support is performed.

Rationale for High-Dose Therapy

Hryniuk and Bush hypothesized the importance of dose intensity in 1984 to examine the effectiveness of various CMF regimens in metastatic breast cancer [2]. Results of three different dose intensities of CAF chemotherapy from the recently completed Cancer and Leukaemia Group B (CALGB) 8541 trial revealed a dose-response relationship in node-positive breast cancer further supporting this concept [3]. Some studies of dose intensity have not demonstrated the same relationship, e.g. the NSABP B-22 trial did not demonstrate a dose-response relationship in the adjuvant trial of primary breast cancer between 600 and 1200 mg/m^2 of cyclophosphamide.

Dose intensification can be achieved by several means including: 1) increasing the total amount of drug administered over a given period of time (increased AUC), or 2) increasing the rate of delivery such that the peak concentration is higher (C_{max}). These two considerations are not necessarily concordant. Further, for some agents such as the antimetabolites, there may be little or no advantage to dose escalation beyond a certain range. Alkylating agents generally have been used as the primary agents of high-dose chemotherapy. These drugs have a number of properties that make their use in combination attractive. Alkylating agents often differ from each other in the dose-limiting toxicity when the myelosuppression is abrogated by the use of haemopoietic progenitor support.

High-Dose Therapy in Metastatic Breast Cancer

Early experiences with multiple alkylating agents led to a phase II trial of high-dose CPA/cDDP/BCNU as initial treatment for women with metastatic breast cancer which had not been previously treated. Peters et al. demonstrated a CR of 54% and an overall response rate of 77% of all patients treated. The median duration of response for the complete responders was 9 months. With a minimal follow-up of 8 years, 3 of 22 patients (14%) remain in unmaintained complete remission (Fig. 1).

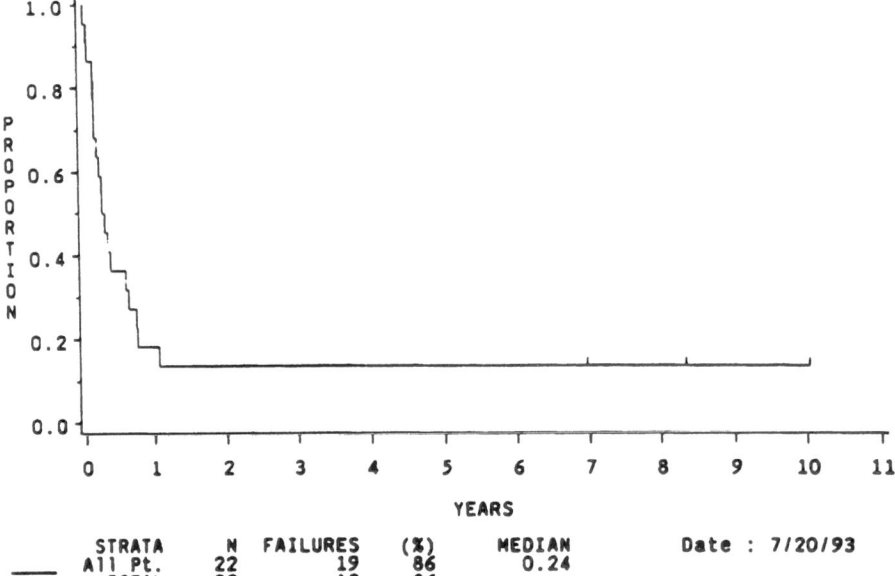

Fig. 1. Long-term event-free survival for women with oestrogen receptor metastatic breast cancer after a single high-dose chemotherapy using cyclophosphamide, cisplatin and BCNU and autologous bone marrow transplantation

Similar results have also been reported in a number of other phase II trials of high-dose chemotherapy [4-7]. To develop a high-dose regimen with good activity in breast and to decrease the transplant-related mortality Antman et al. performed a phase II study of cyclophosphamide, thiotepa and carboplatin with autologous marrow support [4]. Between 1988 and 1992, 62 women with metastatic disease that responded to standard chemotherapy were treated with this regimen. The 5-year DFS for the entire group was 21% (95% confidence interval (CI), 10% to 32%). Patients who were in CR at the time of high-dose chemotherapy had 5-year DFS of 31% (95% CI, 0-63%) [8]. Univariate analysis showed that a single site of disease, CR to induction therapy, prolonged interval from primary diagnosis to first metastases, oestrogen receptor-negative tumours, and age ≥ 40 years were associated with prolonged DFS.

The Autologous Bone Marrow Transplant Registry was established to provide a means of registering and collecting data from multiple institutions and assessing outcomes by pooling of the data. With this method patients are registered by centres, and then detailed case report forms are completed for each patient registered. Unfortunately, the registry data have limited median follow-up at the present time. Although many patients have been registered, complete data are available on only a fraction

of them. Over time, however, the registry may prove to be an important source of collective information. This data collection method is particularly important for analysing subtle differences between treatments, stages of disease, or sites of involvement, or even methods of supportive care. The registry has made great efforts to have complete case reports of each of the various aspects of the protocol under which each patient has been treated.

Until recently studies of high-dose chemotherapy for metastatic breast cancer have been single arm, which may bias the results. Bezwoda et al. have reported the results of a clinical trial comparing high-dose chemotherapy with a conventional-dose regimen as primary treatment for women with metastatic breast cancer. They were able to increase the dose intensity for two drugs, cyclophosphamide and mitoxantrone, 3.8 and 2.2-fold respectively, without encountering dose-limiting toxicity. The high-dose regimen was significantly better than the conventional-dose regimen. The CR was 51% versus 4%, and the overall response rates were 96% and 53%, respectively (Table 1).

In 1988, The Duke Bone Marrow Transplant Program initiated a prospective, randomised trial of high-dose therapy in patients with metastatic breast cancer (Fig. 2). Patients had to have histologically demonstrated, measurable metastatic breast cancer. Patients' tumours

Table 1. Response to treatment

	High-dose CNV		CNV	
	Number	(%)	Number	(%)
CR	23/45	(51)	2/45	(4) *
PR	20/45	(44)	22/45	(49)
PD	2/45	(4)	21/45	(47)

* p < 0.01
Source [13]

were required to be hormone receptor negative or to have demonstrated progression on hormonal therapy. Patients received induction chemotherapy with doxorubicin, fluorouracil and methotrexate (AFM). A maximum of 4 cycles was administered for a lifetime doxorubicin exposure of 500 mg/m^2 or until evidence that further tumour regression had stopped. Patients obtaining CR were randomised to either consolidation therapy with high-dose CPB or to observation. Patients in the observation group were offered high-dose therapy and autologous transplant at the time of recurrence. Patients achieving PR were offered high-dose chemotherapy and transplantation in an effort to convert these patients to CR. A preliminary report of this data has been presented in abstract form and indicated a tripling of the EFS for patients treated with high-dose chemotherapy as consolidation. Interestingly, the strategy of using a transplant at the time of recurrence after CR gave a better overall survival than high-dose chemotherapy early after CR.

Primary Breast Cancer

The prognosis for women with 10 or more axillary lymph nodes involved at the time of presentation is generally poor. With surgery alone or in combination with radiation therapy only 20-30% of women will be alive and free of disease at 5 years. Adjuvant chemotherapy has improved the DFS and overall survival but 65-70% of women will still relapse [9]. Because of the high rate of recurrence after standard adjuvant chemotherapy in high-risk primary breast

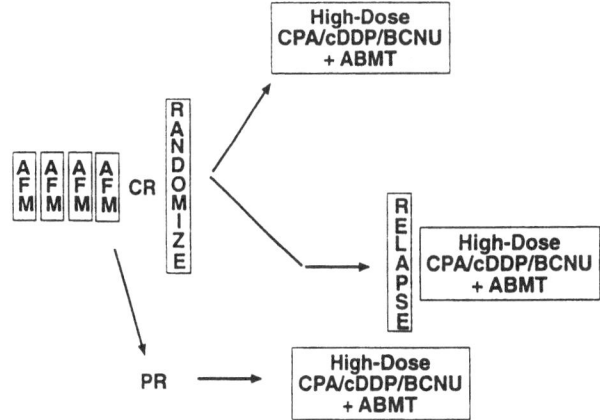

Fig. 2. Treatment schema for AFM trial of high-dose chemotherapy and autologous bone marrow transplantation in women with metastatic breast cancer

cancer, Peters et al. examined the use of high-dose chemotherapy in such patients after standard-dose adjuvant therapy [10]. Eighty-five patients were registered and treated with induction therapy and high-dose chemotherapy. The actual event-free survival (defined as freedom from any local or systemic relapse, early or late therapy-related death) determined by product-limit estimates was 64%, with a median follow-up in excess of 6 years. The overall survival was 72% (95% CI, 64% to 84%). These results are currently being evaluated in a randomised multi-group trial.

As advances in supportive care have occurred the mortality and morbidity of high-dose chemotherapy have decreased. Although the risk of recurrences is slightly lower in women with 4-9 nodes involved than in patients having involvement of 10 or more lymph nodes, 74% will still develop metastatic disease [11]. Two pilot studies have been completed using high-dose chemotherapy in these patients. An intergroup trial involving the South-Western Oncology Group, Eastern Oncology Group, and Cancer and Leukemia Group B will be opened in 1996 to compare high-dose chemotherapy and autologous progenitor cell transplantation with another sequential intensive chemotherapy regimen. Because of the long follow-up required in patients with breast cancer the results of these trials will not be known until early in the twenty-first century.

Conclusion

The definition of the role of high-dose chemotherapy in the management of metastatic and
locally advanced breast cancer has rapidly
progressed over the last 15 years. The data of
phase II studies have provided evidence that
dose-intensification using bone marrow or
PBPC support improves outcome in metastatic
and primary breast cancer. The majority of the
information is based on non-randomised comparisons, and the results of the ongoing randomised trials will be of great importance to
determine the final role of this type of therapy.
The prognosis of breast cancer depends on
many factors, and thus the potential for bias
remains a limitation for any conclusions not
based on a randomised clinical trial design.
Further, the natural history of breast cancer is
long, and extended follow-up of patients enrolled in such trials is essential. The results of a
randomised trial from Bezwoda and colleagues
has provided additional evidence for these
concepts. Other randomised trials are well under way for both primary and metastatic disease, although the results of such trials are
likely to require years of follow-up before being
reported. Until the results of these trials are
available, wherever possible, patients should
be referred to centres participating in the randomised trials; in this way, the more rapid com-
pletion of the trials will be facilitated. Although
the morbidity and mortality of high-dose therapy have been reduced substantially in expe-
rienced hands in the last few years through the
use of PBPC and improved supportive care, it
still carries a 3%-5% mortality. For this reason,
it remains the standard of care that this procedure be restricted to centres with the training
and facilities appropriate to its safe use. Stan-
dards for centres have been adopted by the
American Society of Clinical Oncology and the
American Society of Hematology.
A number of issues remain to be resolved, including the timing of high-dose chemotherapy,
the usefulness, if any, of induction chemotherapy, the importance of residual malignant cells

in the bone marrow or peripheral blood progenitor cell product, defining more effective conditioning regimens, cost-effectiveness and long-
term complication of this form of therapy.
Only 15-30% of patients achieving a complete
remission following high-dose chemotherapy
will remain free of recurrence of their disease.
Relapse may occur because of kinetic resistance of tumour rather than absolute drug resistance. A number of approaches might be effective in overcoming this problem. The use of
sequential high-dose chemotherapy with non-
cross-resistant drugs is being investigated at a
number of centres. The data from the Peters
randomised trail suggest that a delay in high-
dose chemotherapy following induction chemotherapy improves overall survival perhaps by
allowing breast cancer cells to enter the cell
cycle and therefore increase the sensitivity of
alkylating or other chemotherapeutic agents.
An additional reason for treatment failure of
high-dose chemotherapy and autologous haematopoietic progenitor cell transplantation is the
reinfusion of clonogenic malignant cells. With
the use of sensitive immunohistochemical techniques, 19% to 28% of women will have evidence of tumour cells detected at the time of
diagnosis [12]. Peripheral blood progenitors are
frequently used as a source of haematopoietic
progenitor cells after high-dose chemotherapy.
Advantages of PBPC include a more rapid
haematopoietic recovery than after autologous
bone marrow transplantation. One question is
whether tumour cells might also be mobilised
and collected along with the peripheral blood
progenitor cells.
The long-term effects of high-dose therapy are
unknown at this time. The potential complication of second malignancies is unclear, and
careful follow-up of treated populations will be
important. The acute morbidity associated with
high-dose therapy will need to be carefully
monitored. At the present time, the dominant
problem with high-dose therapy, particularly in
the metastatic disease setting, remains relapse.
Nevertheless, long-term toxicity will be of major
importance for the development of this therapeutic approach.

REFERENCES

1   Harris JR, Morrow M, Bonadonna G: Treatment of overt metastatic breast cancer. In: DeVita VT, Hellman S, Rosenberg SA (eds) Cancer: Principles and Practice of Oncology. Lippincott, Philadelphia 1993 pp 1315-1331

2   Hryniuk W and Busch H: The importance of dose intensity in chemotherapy of metastatic breast cancer. J Clin Oncol 1984 (2):1281

3   Wood WC, Budman DR, Korzun AH et al: Dose and dose intensity of adjuvant chemotherapy for stage II, node-positive breast cancer. N Engl J Med 1994 (330):1253

4   Antman K, Ayash L, Elias A et al: A phase II study of high-dose cyclophosphamide, thiotepa, and carboplatin with autologous marrow support in women with measurable advanced breast cancer responding to standard dose therapy. J Clin Oncol 1992 (10):102-110

5   Dunphy FR, Spitzer G, Buzdar AU et al: Treatment of estrogen receptor-negative or hormonally refractory breast cancer with double high-dose chemotherapy intensification and bone marrow support. J Clin Oncol 1990 (7):1207-1216

6   Williams ST, Mick R, Desser R et al: High-dose consolidation therapy with autologous stem cell rescue in stage IV breast cancer. J Clin Oncol 1989 (7): 1824-1830

7   Williams ST, Gilewski T, Mick R et al: High-dose consolidation therapy with autologous stem cell rescue in stage IV breast cancer: follow-up report 1992. J Clin Oncol 1992 (10):1743-1747

8   Ayash LJ, Wheeler C, Fairclough et al: Prognostic factors for prolonged progression-free survival with high-dose chemotherapy with autologous stem-cell support for advanced breast cancer. J Clin Oncol 1995 (13):2043-2049

9   Jones SE, Moon TF, Bonadonna G et al: Comparison of different trials of adjuvant chemotherapy in stage II breast cancer using a nature history database. Am J Clin Oncol 1987 (10):387-395

10 Peters WP, Ross M, Vredenburgh JJ et al: High-dose chemotherapy and autologous bone marrow support as consolidation after standard dose adjuvant therapy for high-risk primary breast cancer. J Clin Oncol 1993 (11):1132-1143

11 Bonadonna G, Valagussa P, Moluterni A, Zambetti M, Brambilla C: Adjuvant cyclophosphamide, methotrexate and fluorouracil in node-positive breast cancer. The results of 20 years of follow-up. N Engl J Med 1995 (332):901-906

12 Diel IJ, Kaufmann M, Goerner R, Costa SC, Kaul S, Bastert G: Detection of tumor cells in bone marrow of patients with primary breast cancer: A prognostic factor for distant metastases. J Clin Oncol 1992 (10):1534-1539

13 Bezwoda WR, Seymour L, Dansey RD: High-dose chemotherapy with hematopoietic rescue as primary treatment for metastatic breast cancer: a randomised trial. J Clin Oncol 1995 (13):2483-2489

Multiple Alkylating Agent Chemotherapy for Solid Cancers

Robert C.F. Leonard

Department of Clinical Oncology, Western General Hospital, Crewe Road, Edinburgh EH4 2XU, Scotland

This chapter examines the evidence for the use of multiple alkylating agent chemotherapy in advanced solid cancers. In clinical research there is an accumulating body of data on human breast cancer, with a much smaller number of studies being pursued in ovarian cancer, small cell lung cancer and testicular cancer. The data from studies of dose intensity within the standard range in advanced breast cancer and in the adjuvant setting have been examined elsewhere and will not be considered further here [1-3].

Theoretical Considerations

The prerequisite for curative drug therapy in any human malignancy is the achievement of complete clinical remission. There is little doubt that such evidence as is currently available supports the concept of intensive chemotherapy as the most effective means of achieving complete remission in relatively chemosensitive but incurable advanced cancer such as breast cancer. Intensive chemotherapy is defined here as an intensity of treatment above that normally achieved because of the use of specific support treatments to overcome potentially lethal myelotoxicity.

Within the context of intensive chemotherapy there is a debate between protagonists for the simple, single high-dose treatment to consolidate remission following induction therapy at standard doses and - increasingly - the use of more than one high-dose treatment supported by progenitor cell infusions, not necessarily preceded by conventional dose induction. Both of these strategies are supported by sound hypotheses [4-8]. The rate of tumour regression is proportional to tumour growth rate and to drug dose, with the former related inversely to tumour size [9]. This suggests that late intensification should succeed. However, the very propensity for rapid regrowth in small tumours makes them difficult to eradicate and suggests the potential for the different strategy of short intervals of intensive therapy, possibly even earlier in treatment [10].

A single high dose of chemotherapy produces a complete response in about 50% of advanced breast cancer where there has been no previous chemotherapy for metastatic disease. Approximately 25% of these complete remissions have been reported to be continuous beyond 5 years [11-30]. The protagonists for multiple high-dose regimens argue that the first condition required for curative therapy, that of complete response, has been achieved but that theoretical and clinical observations in curable cancers suggest that a single dose cannot be adequate and that the situation in metastatic breast cancer parallels that of metastatic curable lymphoma or testis cancer, which is that even in these chemosensitive diseases more than one effective pulse of chemotherapy is required to convert from complete response to a high rate of cure.

Laboratory Studies

Dose Response

The antitumour effect of cytotoxic agents varies with dose, tumour type and agent. Few compounds show such a convincing dose-response characteristic as the classical alkylating agents. The dose-response effect applies to a variety of tumour types including breast cancer cell lines and xenografts of breast cancer cell lines in rodents. The increments in dose seen in these experiments mimic the level of dose increment that can be achieved in the clinic [3,8].

Alkylating Agents - Dose Escalation

For some compounds the dose ratio that can be achieved is impressive, at up to 30-fold increment for thiotepa, but for most other alkylating agents the levels can be escalated to only 4-10 fold above conventional levels before lethal second organ toxicity reaches unacceptable rates. For some compounds the dose increment achievable seems suboptimal, being only 1.5-3 fold in the cases of cisplatin or mitomycin C [3,6,8].

Among the theoretical objections to dose increment above a certain level is the potential for saturating activation systems for some compounds which are prodrugs, e.g. the alkylating oxazophorines. However, allowing for some uncertainty about ifosfamide there is no strong evidence for this as a real problem. Conversely, there is no evidence that the detoxification processes become saturated with the result that toxicity is largely predictable.

Resistance to Alkylators

Importantly, it seems difficult to induce high levels of resistance to alkylating agents in cell lines. Typically, 3-15 fold levels of resistance are achievable as against 5-30 fold increments in dose. Also the limited number of available studies indicates that cross-resistance between different classes of alkylators is weak or absent [3,4].

Multiple Alkylating Agents

Skipper's work on cell lines suggested that a spontaneous rate of mutation which could produce resistance to a given anticancer compound is of the order of 10^{-5} to 10^{-6}. Manifest cancer and even subclinical disease (as in the adjuvant setting) is thus theoretically incurable with a single agent. The problem arises of how much can be compromised on the dose curve of that achievable with the single agent by adding a second or third agent to overcome this frequency of resistance. Assuming that three agents have equivalent but discrete anticancer activity, it is a simple matter of addition to calculate the relative impact of three drugs given at suboptimal doses compared to one or two at optimal dose.

This begs the question of what is clinically achievable due to second organ effects in man that are not predicted from the laboratory. Also the issue of whether the drugs should be given simultaneously or in a compressed schedule over a few days is important. It is in this area of detail that laboratory models begin to break down and the question is left to the clinician to solve.

Multiple High Dose Chemotherapy - Clinical Experience

Spitzer and colleagues at the MD Anderson Cancer Center were early protagonists for dual or "tandem" high-dose chemotherapy in metastatic breast cancer [17]. Using sub-ablative intensification after remission induction they combined two alkylating agents, cisplatin and cyclophosphamide, with etoposide and reported a 50% complete remission rate with 14% durable remission at 5 years of follow-up.

Increasing the intensity of therapy to myeloablative levels soon produced more difficulties. Pittman and colleagues reported a high rate of fatal pulmonary toxicity in patients who had received two successive doses of intensive chemotherapy [18]. Similarly in a series of metastatic breast cancers treated at the Memorial Hospital, Crown and colleagues reported a high rate of non-haematological toxicity following a regimen involving two doses of cyclophosphamide delivered at 14-day intervals followed by a combination regimen of carboplatinum, cyclophosphamide and etoposide in patients already in clinical remission following chemotherapy, radiotherapy or combination [19]. This was a small series of only 17 patients. The cyclophosphamide dosing required no progenitor cell support being given at 3 grams per square metre but, supported by G-CSF, it was used to enhance the yield of the progenitor cell harvest to support the triple high-dose regimen. Follow-up was too short to report on duration but in 5 patients with assessable disease, 2 converted from PR to CR lasting at 10 months of follow-up. Despite non-haematological toxicity, there were no treatment-associated deaths. In a subsequent series the intensity of chemotherapy was increased further with the production of an impressive sustained complete remission rate. Unfortunately the cost in terms of treatment-induced mortality was unacceptable and has prompted a reconsideration of the basic design that incorporates lessons learned from the first two series of studies. However, the principle of progenitor-supported multiple high-dose pulsed chemotherapy remains as the basic design.

At other institutions, a degree of compromise has been adopted in attempts to follow a tandem design. One incorporates a single dose of cyclophosphamide 4-7 g/m^2 that, boosted by G-CSF, mobilises PBPC used to support the subsequent multi-agent myeloablative treatment.

The most commonly used agents are thiotepa and cyclophosphamide, sometimes supplemented by carboplatinum or sometimes incorporating melphalan.

Data from Edinburgh are typical of the current studies in advanced breast cancer. Patients who responded to a non-alkylating induction regimen comprising doxorubicin 20-25 mg/m^2 weekly and infused 5-fluorouracil at 200 mg/m^2 daily for 12 weeks were given high-dose cyclophosphamide 4 g/m^2 followed by G-CSF, progenitor cell harvesting and then thiotepa 125 mg/m^2 daily for 4 days followed by melphalan 140 mg/m^2. This produced a high remission rate converting the induction CR rate from 20% to 55%. There were no treatment-induced

deaths and about 15% remain in continuous CR up to 3 years from intensification. However, the true impact of such treatment remains to be determined as inevitable patient selection effects have to be allowed for in all uncontrolled studies.

One glimmer of insight has recently appeared in a randomised trial reported by Bezwoda et al. [20]. In this trial conventional doses of mitrozantrone, cyclophosphamide and vincristine (6 courses) were compared to mitrozantrone, cyclophosphamide and etoposide at high doses repeated 6 weeks later. Of 45 patients randomised to high dose only 36 received 2 doses, 5 refused and 4 had prolonged myelosuppression. There is a substantial benefit for tandem high-dose therapy from this trial but the true impact of the randomisation is muddied by the policy of giving adjuvant tamoxifen only to those patients in complete remission, thus potentially accentuating the high-dose effect in a cohort of patients which included 27% ER-positive disease in the high-dose arm.

A summary of clinical research based on fully published reports is shown in Table 1 [17-30].

Adjuvant Trials

The results of Peters' study of intensification in the adjuvant treatment of very poor risk breast cancer have encouraged American and other collaborative groups to set up randomised trials [31-33]. The best designs should surely compare best standard therapy against optimal high-dose chemotherapy. This is not easy to

Table 1. Strategies and outcomes for high dose in metastatic breast cancer

Average results (single arm studies)	Complete response rate
Salvage	25%
Initial	50%
Consolidation	60-70%
Randomised trial	
Bezwoda et al. (tandem high dose)	51% (conventional arm 4%)
Median disease-free survival	80 weeks vs 34 weeks (conventional)
Median overall survival	90 weeks vs 45 weeks (conventional)

achieve given the uncertainty about what constitutes best conventional therapy. Many have simply settled on some form of anthracycline combination as best standard treatment. It will be a pity if in 5 years' time high-dose therapy, whether in single or multiple pulses, is merely proved better than inadequate standard treatment.

Carcinoma of the Ovary

As in breast cancer there are data from preclinical studies and from clinical research within the standard dose range to support the concept of dose intensity influencing survival in advanced ovarian cancer.

Dose-Intensive Studies

As in early trials in breast cancer many of the myeloablative regimens incorporated drugs that were capable of escalation, being predictably myelotoxic but not necessarily of proven benefit against the tumour under study. However, overall response rates above 60% in studies incorporating patients with known refractory and/or relapsed disease supported the idea of a real dose-response effect. The cost has been one of morbidity and treatment-induced mortality and at present high-dose chemotherapy using alkylating or other agents cannot be recommended for early relapse or resistant disease. This may not be the situation, however, for late relapse; in these patients, and particularly in those in first remission with poor long-term prognosis due to adverse presentational features, there is some interest in examining high-dose chemotherapy in trials [34-36].

Testicular Cancer

Initial studies of intensive chemotherapy were carried out in refractory and relapsed disease (a miscellaneous group) in a manner analogous to most other disease types. A cure rate of 10-20% has encouraged further research incorporating known active alkylators, cyclophosphamide and carboplatinum with etoposide. However, the results in truly refractory disease are poor, with treatment-induced mortality of 10-

20% and few cures. Studies have been conducted in first relapse using single and double transplants, the latter facilitated by progenitor cell support. A study of 21 patients with poor prognosis disease which included 6 incomplete responders and 15 in relapse produced 67% DFS at 3 years' median follow-up, the high-dose regimen combining either carboplatin 1200 mg/m^2; etoposide 3 g/m^2 and ifosfamide 6 g/m^2 or carboplatin 800 mg/m^2; etoposide 2.4 g/m^2 and cyclophosphamide 7.2 g/m^2 followed by ABMT. Similar results using similar regimens in comparable patients have been reported elsewhere. Data from Memorial Hospital support the idea of initial high-dose chemotherapy similar to their research in breast cancer. At present it seems that dose intensification of about 50% above standard doses can be delivered safely, with the outcome of improved durable response rates. However, controlled trial data are lacking. Due to the inherent rarity and predictably small benefits, it will be a slow task to complete the randomised trials that could prove such benefits [37,38].

Small Cell Lung Cancer

A decade ago this was the lead cancer for study of late intensification. However, the studies could all be criticised for their design: many were small scale, all suffered from patient attrition between induction and presentation for dose escalation and nearly all were uncontrolled "pilot" studies. The current perception, however, is that SCLC is a basically refractory disease and there is limited enthusiasm for trials of dose intensification, even allowing for the fact that one or two new agents such as carboplatinum have become available since the last spate of studies [39,40].

Conclusions

There is growing public as well as medical interest in the use of intensive chemotherapy in some of the solid cancers. In advanced breast cancer there is particular interest in the potential for multiple high-dose chemotherapy to improve on the tantalising data indicating durable remission in a small proportion of patients treated with a single high-dose combination.

In this as well as other cancers, the pragmatic and theoretical advantages of alkylating agents make them the mainstay of most combination regimens. The debate about combination versus single-agent high-dose treatment seemingly favours combination regimens, albeit without the proof of randomised comparisons. Even with the data from Bezwoda's study, the place of double or multiple or even single high-dose chemotherapy is by no means established in breast cancer. Randomised trials are under way in advanced disease and in poor-risk patients in the adjuvant setting.

The place of multiple alkylator intensification in other tumour types is even less established although there seems to be a real benefit for the few poor-risk teratoma patients. Whether trials can be done to clarify the position of high-dose chemotherapy outside breast cancer remains to be seen, but it will undoubtedly take some years of carefully planned and executed collaborative research to achieve an answer [41-44].

REFERENCES

1   Henderson IC, et al: Cancer of the Breast. In: De-Vita VT, Hellman S, Rosenberg SA (eds) Cancer: Principles and Practice of Oncology. JB Lippincott, Philadelphia 1989 pp 1197-1268
2   Early Breast Cancer Trialists' Collaborative Group: Systemic treatment of early breast cancer by hormonal, cytotoxic or immune therapy: 133 randomised trials involving 31000 recurrences and 24000 deaths among 75000 women. Lancet 1992 (339):1-5; 71-85
3   DeVita VT: Principles of chemotherapy. In: DeVita VT, Hellman S, Rosenberg SA (eds) Cancer: Principles and Practice of Oncology, 4th edition. JB Lippincott, Philadelphia 1983
4   Skipper H: Data and analyses having to do with the influence of dose intensity and duration of treatment (single drug combinations) on lethal toxicity and therapeutic response of experimental neoplasms. Southern Research Institute, Birmingham Booklets 13 1986 and 2-13 1987
5   Antmann K: Dose-intensive chemotherapy in breast cancer. In: Armitage J and Antmann K (eds) High Dose Cancer Therapy. Pharmacology, Haemopoietins, Stem Cells. Williams and Wilkins, Baltimore 1992
6   Teicher B, Cucchi C, Lee J et al: Alkylating agents. Studies of cross resistance. Patterns in human tumor cell lines. Cancer Res 1987 (46):4379-4383
7   Norton L: Synopsis of cell kinetics and cancer chemotherapy. In: Silver RT (ed) Handbook of Cancer Chemotherapy, 2nd edition. Little and Brown, Boston 1987
8   Frei E, Cucchi C, Rosowsky A et al: Alkylating agent resistance: in vitro studies with human cell lines. Proc Natl Acad Sci USA 1985 (82):2158-2162
9   Norton L: A Compertzian model of human breast cancer growth. Cancer Res 1988 (48):7067-7071
10   Crown J and Norton L: Potential strategies for improving the results of high-dose chemotherapy in patients with metastatic breast cancer. Ann Oncol 1995 (6 Suppl 4):S21-S26
11   Eddy DM: High-dose chemotherapy with autologous bone marrow transplantation for the treatment of metastatic breast cancer. J Clin Oncol 1992 (10): 657-670
12   Triozzi PL: Autologous bone marrow and peripheral blood progenitor transplant for breast cancer. Lancet 1994 (344): 418-419
13   Leonard RCF: High dose chemotherapy for metastatic breast cancer. Lancet 1994 (344):1084
14   Frei E, Antmann K, Teicher B et al: Bone marrow autotransplantation for solid tumours - Prospects. J Clin Oncol 1989 (7):515-526
15   Antmann KH and Souhami RL: High dose chemotherapy in solid tumours. A review of published data in selected tumours with a commentary. Ann Oncol 1993 (Suppl 1):539-544
16   Thomas ED: Hemopoietic stem cell transplantation. Science Medicine 1995 (2):38-47
17   Lazarus H, Reed MD, Spitzer TR et al: High-dose iv thiotepa and cryopreserved autologous bone mar-row transplantation for therapy of refractory cancer. Cancer Treat Rep 1987 (71):689-695
18   Pittman KL, To LB, Bayly JL et al: Non-haematological toxicity limiting the application of sequential high-dose chemotherapy in patients with advanced breast cancer. Bone Marrow Transplant 1992 (10): 535-540
19   Crown J, Kritz A, Vahdat L et al: Rapid administration of multiple cycles of high dose myelosuppressive chemotherapy in patients with metastatic breast cancer. J Clin Oncol 1993 (11):1144-1149
20   Bezwoda WR, Seymour L, Dansey RD: High-dose chemotherapy with hematopoietic rescue as primary treatment for metastatic breast cancer: a randomised trial. J Clin Oncol 1995 (13):2483-2489
21   Ghallie R, Richman CM, Adler SA et al: Treatment of metastatic breast cancer with a split-course high-dose chemotherapy regimen and autologous bone marrow transplantation. J Clin Oncol 1994 (12):342-346
22   Dunphy F, Spitzer G, Rossiter-Fornoff JE et al: Factors predicting long-term survival for metastatic breast cancer patients treated with high-dose chemotherapy and bone marrow support. Cancer 1994 (73):2157-2167
23   Kennedy MJ, Beveridge RA, Rowley SD Gordon GB, Abeloff MD, Davidson NE: High dose chemotherapy with reinfusion of purged autologous bone marrow following dose intense induction as initial therapy for metastatic breast cancer. JNCI 1991 (83):920-926
24   Mulder NH, Mulder POM, Sleijfer DT et al: Induction chemotherapy and intensification with autologous bone marrow reinfusion in patients with locally advanced and disseminated breast cancer. Eur J Cancer 1993 (29A):668-671
25   Ayash L, Elias A, Wheeler C et al: Double dose-intensive chemotherapy with autologous marrow and peripheral-blood progenitor-cell support for metastatic breast cancer. J Clin Oncol 1994 (12): 37-44
26   Coiffier B, Philip T, Burnett AK, Syman ML: Consensus conference on intensive chemotherapy plus hematopoietic stem-cell transplantation in malignancies: Lyon, France, June 4-6 1993. J Clin Oncol 1994 (12):226-231
27   Sledge GW Jr and Antman KH: Progress in chemotherapy for metastatic breast cancer. Sem Oncol 1992 (19):317-332
28   Patrone F, Ballestrero A, Ferrando F et al: Four-step high dose sequential chemotherapy with double haematopoietic progenitor-cell rescue for metastatic breast cancer. J Clin Oncol 1995 (13): 840-846
29   Crown J, Wasserheit C, Hakes T et al: Rapid delivery of multiple courses of high dose chemotherapy with granulocyte colony-stimulating factor and peripheral blood derived hematopoietic progenitor cells. JNCI 1992 (84):1935-1936
30   Vahdat L, Raptis G, Fennelly D: Rapidly cycled courses of high-dose alkylating agents supported by filgastrim and peripheral blood progenitor cells in patients with metastastic breast cancer. Clin Cancer Res 1995 (1):1267-1273
31   Peters W, Vredenburgh J, Shpall EJ et al: High dose chemotherapy and autologous bone marrow support

as consolidation after standard dose adjuvant therapy for high risk primary breast cancer. J Clin Oncol 1993 (11):1132-1143

32 Gianni A, Valagusa P, Bonadonna G et al: Growth factor supported high dose chemotherapy in breast cancer with more than 10 nodes. Proc ASCO 1993 (11):60

33 de Graaf H, Willemse P, de Vries E et al: Intensive chemotherapy with autologous bone marrow transfusion as primary treatment of women with breast cancer and more than five involved axillary lymph nodes. Eur J Cancer 1994 (30A):150-153

34 Fennelly D, Schneider J, Spriggs D et al: Dose-escalation of taxol with high-dose cyclophosphamide, with analysis of progenitor cell mobilisation and haematologic support of advanced ovarian cancer patients receiving rapidly sequenced high-dose carboplatin/cyclophosphamide courses. J Clin Oncol 1995 (13):1160-1166

35 Viens P and Maraninchi D: High dose chemotherapy and autologous marrow transplantation for common epithelial ovarian carcinoma. In: Antmann K and Armitage J (eds) High Dose Cancer Therapy. Williams and Wilkins, Baltimore 1992

36 Mainwaring PN and Gore ME: The importance of dose and schedule in cancer chemotherapy: epithelial ovarian cancer. Anticancer Drugs 1995 (Suppl 5): 29-41

37 De Mulder PHM and de Wit R: Experience with dose and schedule variations in germ cell tumours. Anticancer Drugs 1995 (Suppl 5):43-52

38 Broun ER and Nichols CR: High-dose chemotherapy in the management of malignant germ cell tumours. In: Antmann K and Armitage J (eds) High Dose Cancer Therapy. Williams and Wilkins, Baltimore 1992

39 Spitzer G, Spencer V, Dunphy FR: High dose chemotherapy with autologous bone marrow support for lung cancer. In: Antmann K and Armitage J (eds) High Dose Cancer Therapy. Williams and Wilkins, Baltimore 1992

40 Ranson M and Thatcher N: The importance of dose and schedule in chemotherapy for small cell lung cancer. Anticancer Drugs 1995 (Suppl 5):53-63

41 Shea TC, Mason JR, Storniolo AM et al: Sequential cycles of high-dose carboplatin administered with recombinant human granulocyte-macrophage colony-stimulating factor and repeated infusions of autologous peripheral-blood progenitor cells: A novel and effective method for delivering multiple courses of dose-intensive therapy. J Clin Oncol 1992 (10):464-473

42 Tepler I, Cannistra S, Frei E et al: Use of peripheral blood progenitor cells abrogates the myelotoxicity of repetitive high-dose carboplatin and cyclophosphamide chemotherapy. J Clin Oncol 1993 (11): 1583-1592

43 Gianni AM, Siena S, Bregni M et al: Granulocyte-macrophage colony stimulating factor to harvest circulating haematopoietic stem cells for auto-transplantation. The Lancet 1989 (2):580-585

44 Canellos GP: High-dose therapy: Here to stay or just visiting. J Clin Oncol 1994 (12):1-5

The Health Economics of High-Dose Chemotherapy

Matti S. Aapro [1,2] and Franco Nolé [2]

1   Institut Multidisciplinaire d'Oncologie, 1272 Genolier, Switzerland
2   Division of Medical Oncology, European Institute of Oncology, via Ripamonti 435, 20141 Milan, Italy

The economic evaluation of health care has become very popular over the past decade. Many factors could explain the profusion of literature on health economics (HE) in the last few years, but the main reason is that for many diseases more than one clinically acceptable treatment option is available [1]. The different treatment options are, however, not equally affordable nor is there a guarantee of better clinical success proportional to the increase in cost per treatment selected. Therefore choices must be made based on the potential clinical benefit of new treatments balanced against the obtainable budget. HE aids in this evaluation by including in the analysis highly diverse variables such as cost and clinical outcome [2].

Governments today struggle with tight budget constraints, particularly in the loss-making social security sector that includes health care. Over the past decade the national authorities have been confronted with annual increases in total health care costs above the rate of inflation, which can partially be explained by variables like epidemiology, demography, the number of health care providers available on the market, and the number of people covered by compulsory insurance [3].

In order to limit these increases various economy measures are applied such as prospective payment systems, disease-related group (DRG) based payment for each intervention performed, the introduction of formularies for hospital drugs, or the application of generalised co-payment systems. The purpose of these cost-controlling techniques is to make the public-funded benefits correspond to perceived public needs and therefore get 'value for money' [4].

A last step in introducing rational budget management in health care is a thorough application of the analytical techniques developed by HE, as has been recently endorsed by countries like Australia and Canada. The Australian and Canadian authorities require submission of the results of the economic evaluation of new pharmaceuticals to guide Medicare decisions about drug reimbursement [5].

Nevertheless some problems remain. An actual dilemma exists for the medical community when it comes to introducing HE notions in the decision-making process of prescribing drugs or new treatment techniques [6]. Should physicians, by moral or legal obligation, apply all available means to treat a patient when the health care administration tends to restrain the requests put forward by the health care providers? It becomes essential to properly inform and educate the medical community about the benefits of using HE analysis as an important added tool in the medical decision-making process.

This chapter deals with the specific issue of HE related to high-dose chemotherapy (HDC) in cancer treatment. It should provide some guidelines for the medical community. It will support research aimed at evaluating the clinical benefits to be expressed as quality-adjusted life years (QALYs) gained.

While HDC entails increased expenses due to the utilisation of more cytotoxic drugs with an increased risk of toxicities, HE analysis will allow a better appreciation of the medical decisions taken by balancing the extra cost against the extra clinical benefit obtained. In a context of continuous budget cuts for health care, omitting the use of HE evaluation methods might lead to unreasonable decisions being taken for the community.

Medical Cost Evaluation

Physicians are constantly making choices about treatment options to be used. They rely on facts they have been taught, or on evidence gleaned from the medical literature. Unfortunately, many have not been informed about the principles of cost-benefit analyses during their training. Intuitively they apply an equation that balances human suffering against health care benefits, the latter expressed as an improvement in the patient's health status. In order to better quantify this comparison physicians and nurses need to understand the importance of well-performed quality-of-life (QoL) studies. They need to appreciate that QoL instruments developed for such evaluations will demonstrate added value in clinical management and hence in HE analysis [7].

In the future when making their therapeutic choices physicians will be confronted with a new variable: the cost of a particular treatment. Regarding the latter, society has to decide what is financially affordable based on collective measures and the effect on the individual patient's outcome.

There are two main difficulties in performing health economic evaluations [8]. One is to obtain reliable data including the exact perspective of analysis, the type of cost data to be considered and the appropriate clinical outcome variables (Table 1). The other is the right interpretation of the results after the analysis. A sensitivity analysis must be performed on those variables that are subject to variation.

Fortunately authorities in many countries have now developed guidelines on how to conduct HE studies. These guidelines seek to harmonise the principles on which HE evaluations should be based [9].

However, before starting such an analysis, it is important to understand the definitions of the different kinds of HE studies one can apply in particular to HDC. The importance of a rigorous approach to economic evaluation in cancer care has been highlighted in a recent report of the European School of Oncology [10].

Cost-minimisation analysis can only be applied if no difference in effect is observed. It simply compares the cost of two treatment options considered.

Cost-effectiveness analysis compares, besides the cost, the effect of interventions in terms of a common unit, e.g. life years saved. It does not include aspects of QoL-related effects in addition to cost.

In *cost-utility analysis* the effectiveness of the treatment is measured in quality-adjusted life years, whereas in *cost-benefit analysis* the effectiveness is valued in monetary terms, which allows the calculation of net financial gains or losses.

In the case of HDC a simple cost comparison with conventional chemotherapy treatment is not worth performing, because HDC will always be more expensive as the treatment demands a greater use of cytotoxic drugs and presents a higher risk of toxicity, which may require treatment or even preventative measures. However, a simple cost comparison could be appropriate when two HD techniques are compared, for example autologous bone marrow transplant (ABMT) and peripheral blood progenitor cell transplant (PBPCT).

Table 1. Different variables playing a role in HE analysis

Type	Examples*
Perspective	Society, Ministry of Health, hospital, ward, patient
Costs	Real costs, charges, fees, tariffs
- Direct medical cost	Laboratory tests, diagnostic tests, hotel costs, drugs, surgical interventions
- Indirect medical cost	Overhead costs, laundry, cleaning, administration
- Direct non-medical cost	Transport, nutrition
- Indirect non-medical cost	Sick leave
Outcome results	Mortality, disease-free survival (DFS), morbidity, QoL, QALYs

*the list is not exhaustive

The relevant economic issue in HDC as opposed to standard-dose chemotherapy is to consider if the increased clinical effectiveness of HDC compensates for its added marginal costs. Moreover, HDC is delivered in a shorter period of time compared to conventional-dose chemotherapy because higher dose intensity is sought at the expense of more potential toxicities. Therefore it would be valuable to carry out an in-depth analysis of QoL changes over time during treatment and to evaluate the differences in indirect cost when the patient can recover more promptly after HDC.

Budget Expenditure on Cancer Treatment

Cost containment in cancer care can be applied in many different ways. It may range from a rational use of laboratory tests and other diagnostic features, such as radiological facilities, to the adequate prescription of anticancer therapy.

Two numerical examples are presented here, which may help to understand the potential impact of cost containment within cancer care on the total health care budget of a country.

The health care budget in the United Kingdom runs close to 75 billion US dollars a year (1996). However, the annual expenditure for cancer treatment accounts for only 3% of this total budget, despite the fact that cancer is the second cause of mortality in the UK. Of that cancer budget, only 3% is devoted to chemo-

therapy. The latter figure may be compared to the same amount of money spent on laxatives or anti-acne treatment in this country [11].

Data from 1992 available for Switzerland indicate that with its 6.9 million inhabitants the country spent 22.4 billion US dollars on public health, of which 51% were used for in-hospital care, 38.2% for out-patient care and 7.3% for drugs (with an unreported proportion for cytotoxic drugs). The remaining amount (3.5%) was spent on various other items. In the same year 27.2% of all deaths among the Swiss population were due to cancer. By contrast, only 9 million US dollars were spent on out-patient chemotherapy, representing only 0.4% of all drugs prescribed for ambulatory care [12].

Moreover, the often claimed high costs of cancer treatment have been frequently overemphasized by skeptics saying that cancer treatment, with a few exceptions, is of little proven benefit [13].

The current cost impact of cancer treatment on society may be deduced from the above considerations. This is a partial view of the problem and may suggest that the cost of drug treatment in cancer patients is not as excessive as so often reported. A more objective way to compare cost of treatment figures for different disease groups is to evaluate treatment interventions in terms of cost per life year saved, as shown in Table 2 [14]. It is obvious from such a comparison that some undisputed approaches in medicine - but also in oncology - should better justify their real cost.

Table 2. Cost-effectiveness ratios in some oncological and non-oncological situations

Intervention	Cost/life year (US $)
Routine carcinoembryonic antigen monitoring after colon cancer	31,000-6,600,000
Adjuvant CMF for breast cancer patient aged 45 years	4,900
ABMT for limited metastatic breast carcinoma	115,800
Coronary artery bypass	106,000
Treatment of hypertension	23,500

costs in US dollars, 1992
Modified from [14]

Cost-Minimisation Studies in High-Dose Chemotherapy

The following two examples show the application of cost-minimisation analysis that has supported the introduction of new treatment techniques and new drugs in HDC.

The first example concerns the comparison of ABMT with PBPCT. Many recent articles have presented results which compare the direct medical costs of both techniques [15-18]. All publications show remarkable cost reductions of up to 15-20% with PBPCT. The cost reductions are mainly tangible in the post-transplant period and are related to the reduction of hospital stay, blood product support and infective episodes to be treated.

An interesting feature that becomes apparent following a more in-depth analysis of all the data reported by the different studies is de-

picted in Figure 1. The figure plots on the x-axis the mean cost of PBPCT, expressed in a common currency (US dollars 1996), and on the y-axis the cost difference with the comparator. A linear relationship is observed between both variables, proportional to the mean cost of PBPCT. Surprisingly, one study result does not fit the constructed regression line [15]. It reports a high "cost-difference" discrepancy of up to 30% compared to the other study results. To explain the irregularity one must look at the data as it was originally reported. This study turned out to be the first to compare the two techniques. The investigators failed at that time to properly randomise their mixed patient population of solid and haematological cancers over the two treatment arms. It is important to avoid a potential bias when performing a cost comparative study as it will result in distorted data that cannot be confirmed by other studies.

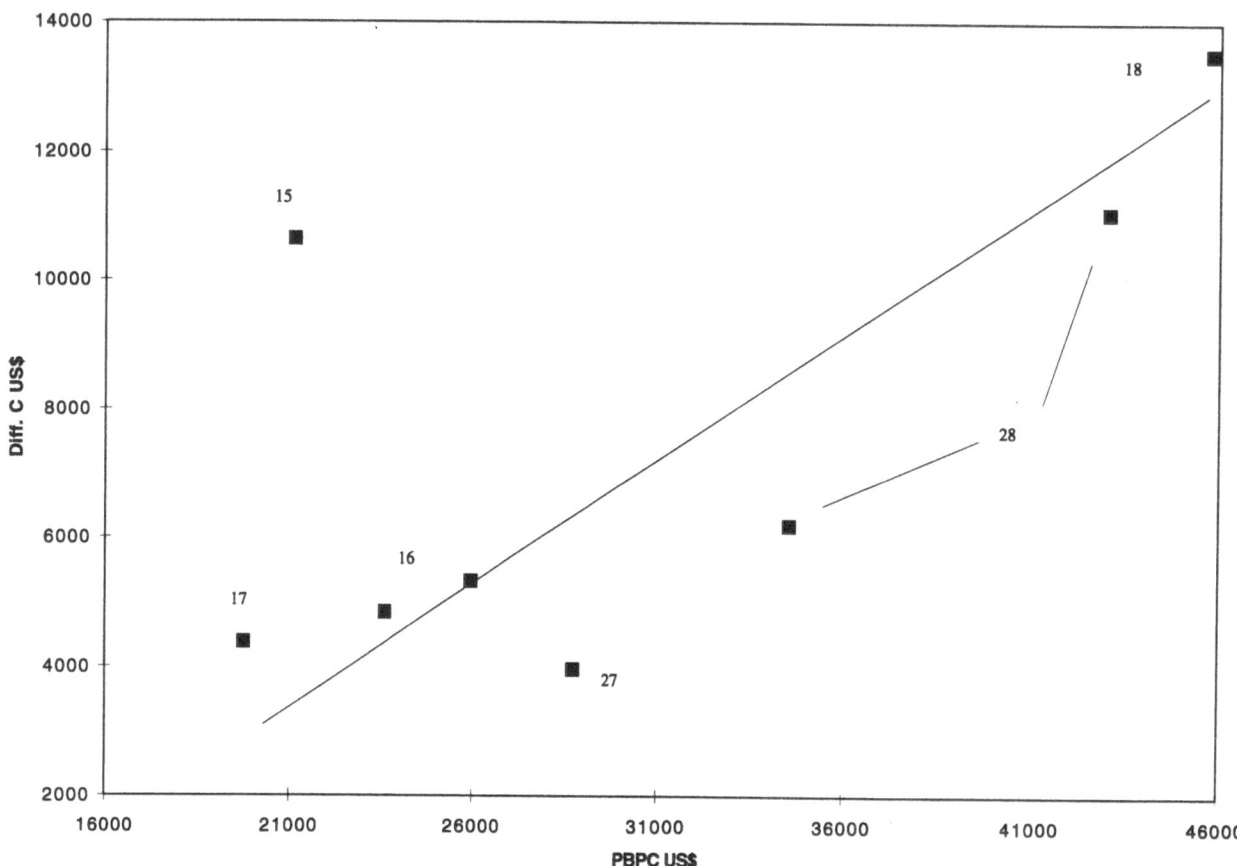

Fig. 1. Cost comparison in US$ of PBPCT (x-axis) and ABMT (y-axis) from different studies [15-18,27,28]

Table 3. Variables to be checked in HE evaluation of different studies comparing PBPCT and ABMT

Type	Specific		
Country	Single/multiple		
Hospital centre	Single/multiple		
Perspective	Hospital, third-party payer, patient, society		
Patient selection	Disease	Stage/Grade	Haematological/Solid
	Age group		
	ECOG performance		
	Autologous/allogeneic		
	Clinical status	PR - CR - PD	
Type of study	Prospective/retrospective		
	Piggyback, No trial		
Study phases	Pre-/post-transfusion		
	Follow-up		
Economic evaluation	Cost comparison		
	Cost-effectiveness	Effect measure	
Unit price calculation	Charges, real cost, tariffs	Currency and year	
Withdrawals	Included, excluded		
Cost variables	Hospitalisation	Normal, Special ward, ICU	
	Outpatient care		
	Drugs	Mobilisation, conditioning, prophylactic	
	Leukapheresis		
	Laboratory tests		
	Diagnostics		
	Transfusion		
	Harvest		
	Toxicities		
	Nutrition		
	BMT intervention		
	Medical consultation		

Table 3 gives a list of variables that need to be checked when a thorough comparison is made between studies on ABMT and PBPCT. Another example where cost-minimisation analysis has been utilised for HDC concerns the human haemopoietic growth factors (granulocyte and granulocyte-macrophage colony stimulating factors, G-CSFs and GM-CSFs). These drugs decrease the neutropenic events induced by myelosuppressive agents and are therefore important in HDC. It has been reported by Lyman in 1993, based on the study results of Crawford, that in the United States cost savings could be obtained by the pro-phylactic use of G-CSF if the incidence rate of febrile neutropenic events was above 40% [19,20]. This analysis included only the direct medical costs in the equation. Recently Lyman suggested that the 40% could be reduced to 20% if the indirect costs were also considered in the analysis [21]. It means that the use of haemopoietic growth factors not only prevents the expensive treatment of a febrile neutropenic event, it also helps patients to remain at work instead of being hospitalised. The drug thus prevents the important additional cost of sick leave.

Table 4. Potential resource impact of haemopoietic growth factors

Resource increase	Effect of HGF	Resource savings
Increased frequency of chemotherapy	Reduced chemotherapy delays	Fewer blood counts Fewer outpatient consultations
More chemotherapy Greater non-myeloid toxicity	Chemotherapy dose escalation	
More outpatient cost?	Reduced risk of infection	Reduced hospital stay Fewer antibiotics Less staff time
	Fewer transfusions	Reduced hospital stay Less use of blood products Less staff time

Reproduced from [22]

Johnson and Rees have demonstrated in their review paper all the potential resource impacts of haemopoietic growth factors (Table 4). It is obvious from this table that the preventative action of haemopoietic growth factors is more complex. It has a wider impact on different resources and hence on costs [22].

Cost-Effectiveness Studies in High-Dose Chemotherapy

As stated before, clinicians, patients and health care purchasers may all have different opinions on the value of a particular therapy. Clinicians and patients are mainly induced to use treatments that improve disease remission or produce survival gains. Budget holders on the other hand will additionally balance cost against clinical gains. Moreover, when working with tight budgets, administrators realise that not all approaches in which the clinical benefit exceeds the costs can be afforded; the treatment showing the highest benefit per cost unit will be preferentially selected in such cases. The latter type of analysis is a cost-effectiveness analysis.

Unfortunately, not many clinical trials in HDC have reported results on cost-effectiveness data, mainly because clinical studies incorporating these measures are a recent phenomenon.

In order to report a meaningful cost-effectiveness result, a sufficiently long follow-up period

should be considered for treatments that potentially lead to cure or show an important rate of disease remission. The longer the survival benefit, the better the cost-effectiveness result will be. Cost-effectiveness data reported after a 3-year follow-up period could therefore look better when reported after 5 years of follow-up when the same survival benefit is observed at the two points in time.

One of the earlier studies presenting cost-effectiveness results of HDC is the article by Bezwoda of 1995 [23,24]. The paper shows that patients with metastatic breast cancer might benefit from high-dose chemotherapy. Table 5 gives the data of the economic analysis performed with the study results. While the initial cost of the HD procedure could be seen as excessive, one has to take into account the demonstrated survival benefit which considerably diminishes the reported "excess" cost.

Finally, over the past decade many researchers have tried to identify quantitative and qualitative methods that better assess the clinical benefits of aggressive chemotherapy. A popular method is the use of QALYs, where the time elapsed between the initiation of a treatment and the end of the follow-up period is valued with an index ranging from 0 (bad QoL) to 1 (perfect QoL) [25].

It has been suggested that, in addition to the clinical gain obtained with HDC, there could be quality-of-life benefits compared with conventional chemotherapy treatment due to the shorter treatment time. This QoL gain could also be considered in the selection of therapeutic op-

Table 5. Cost comparison of high-dose chemotherapy and conventional chemotherapy for metastatic breast cancer

	High-Dose	Conventional
Chemotherapy	7231	5460
Antibiotics	5805	2135
Blood products	4140	255
Hospitalisation	1250	-
Examinations	1736	1468
Growth Factors	5140	-
TOTAL	25282	9318
Mean survival after after 2 years	± 24 months	± 12 months
Cost/life year saved	12651	9318

Costs in South African rands
Reproduced from [24]

tions. Several clinical trials are currently ongoing which analyse this aspect more in depth [26]. In the coming years we are likely to obtain a better insight into the value of QALYs related to HDC.

Conclusions

In the past few years HE assessment and analysis have been used in the evaluation and adoption of new treatment techniques and new drugs, leading to their wider application. The use of HE will also be important with regard to the adoption of HDC and supportive therapies.

PBPCT and G-CSF are two perfect examples in this respect. Their use has increased not only due to their better safety and improved clinical results but also due to the resulting cost savings in some specific situations.

Although the final aim of HE evaluation is to properly associate the clinical outcome results with the cost of resources, very few HE data have been published in the field of HDC, an obviously cost-intensive approach.

In the near future one may expect more cost-effectiveness and possibly cost-utility data to be reported. With the use of these specific analyses HDC treatment could be better evaluated in terms of the extra cost it entails versus the extra clinical benefits it generates compared to other treatments.

It is to be hoped that the HE issue will get due attention not only from the health care budget holders but also from the medical community, which by then will be properly informed about the value of cost-effectiveness analyses.

Acknowledgement

The authors wish to thank Drs B. Standaert, O. Hartmann, R.C.F. Leonard and K. Dupont for their precious help.

REFERENCES

1   Drummond M, Rutten F, Brenna A, Gouveia Pinto C, Horisberger B et al: Economic evaluation of pharmaceuticals. A European perspective. PharmacoEconomics 1993 (4):173-186

2   Drummond M, Stoddart G, Torrance G: Methods for the Economic Evaluation of Health Care Programmes. Oxford Medical Publications. Oxford University Press, 1987

3   Schieber G, Poullier J-P, Greenwald L: US Health Expenditure Performance: An International Comparison and Data Update. Health Care Financing Review. US Department of Health and Human Services, Vol. 13, No. 4, September 1992

4   OECD Health Systems. Facts and Trends 1960-1991, Vol. 1. Health Policy Studies No. 3. OECD, Paris, 1993

5   Jacobs P, Bachynsky J, Baladi J-F: A comparative review of pharmacoeconomic guidelines. PharmacoEconomics 1995 (8):182-189

6   Jonsson V, Clausen SR, Hansen MM: Pharmacoeconomic aspects in the treatment of curable and incurable cancer. PharmacoEconomics 1995 (8): 275-281

7   Drummond M and O'Brien B: Clinical importance, statistical significance and the assessment of economic and quality-of-life outcomes. Health Economics 1993 (2):205-212

8   Bonsel GJ, Rutten F, Uyl-de Groot C: Economic evaluation alongside cancer trials: Methodological and practical aspects. Eur J Cancer 1993 (29A Suppl 7):S10-S14

9   Drummond M: Guidelines for pharmacoeconomic studies. PharmacoEconomics 1994 (6):493-497

10 Williams C, Coyle D, Gray A et al: European School of Oncology advisory report to the Commission of the European Communities for the "Europe against cancer programme" cost-effectiveness in cancer care. Eur J Cancer 1995 (31A):1410-1424

11 Figures quoted by R.C.F. Leonard at a European School of Oncology Task Force meeting, June 1995

12 Ermini M: Public Health in Switzerland. Pharma Information. Basel, 1994

13 Bailar JC and Gornik HL: Cancer undefeated. N Engl J Med 1997 (336):1569-1574

14 Smith TJ, Hillner BE, Desch CE: Efficacy and cost-effectiveness of cancer treatment: rational allocation of resources based on decision analysis. JNCI 1993 (85): 1460-1474

15 Uyl-de Groot C, Richel D, Rutten F: Peripheral blood progenitor cell transplantation mobilised by G-CSF (filgrastim): a less costly alternative to autologous bone marrow transplantation. Eur J Cancer 1994 (30A):1631-1635

16 Hartmann O, Le Corroller A, Blaise D et al: Peripheral blood stem cell and bone marrow transplantation for solid tumors and lymphomas: Hematologic recovery and costs. A randomized, controlled trial. Ann Int Med 1997 (126):600-607

17 Le Corroller A, Faucher C, Auperin A et al: Autologous peripheral blood progenitor cell transplantation versus autologous bone marrow transplantation for adults and children with non-leukaemic malignant disease. A randomised economic study. PharmacoEconomics 1997 (11): 454-463

18 Smith T, Hillner B, Schmitz N et al: Economic analysis of a randomized clinical trial to compare filgrastim-mobilized peripheral blood progenitor cell transplantation and autologous bone marrow transplantation in patients with Hodgkin's and non-Hodgkin's lymphoma. J Clin Oncol 1997 (15): 5-10

19 Crawford J, Ozer H, Stoller R et al: Reduction by granulocyte colony-stimulating factor of fever and neutropenia induced by chemotherapy in patients with small cell lung cancer. N Engl J Med 1991 (315): 164-170

20 Lyman G, Lyman C, Sanderson R, Balducci L: Decision analysis of hematopoietic growth factor use in patients receiving cancer chemotherapy. JNCI 1993 (85):488-493

21 Lyman G, Kuderer N, Green J, Moffit HL: The economics of febrile neutropenia. Blood 1996 (88 Suppl 10): 346a (abstract 1374)

22 Johnson N and Rees G: Economic evaluation of new treatments: haematopoietic growth factors. Clin Oncol 1996 (8):43-47

23 Bezwoda W, Seymour L, Dansey R: High-dose chemotherapy with hematopoietic rescue as primary treatment for metastatic breast cancer: A randomized trial. J Clin Oncol 1995 (13):2483-2489

24 Bezwoda W: High dose chemotherapy in the treatment of breast cancer: Controversies and some answers. Specialist Medicine 1995 (September): 4-14

25 Carr-Hill R and Morris J: Current practice in obtaining the 'Q' in QALYs: A cautionary note. Br Med J 1991 (303):699-701

26 Piccart M and Goldhirsch A: An overview of all the ongoing adjuvant clinical trials for breast cancer in Europe and Canada. Breast International Group

27 Woronoff-Lemsi M, Arveux P, Limat S et al: Cost comparative study of autologous peripheral blood progenitor cells (PBPC) and bone marrow (ABM) transplantation for non-Hodgkin's lymphoma patients. Blood 1995 (86 Suppl 10): 209a (abstract 892)

28 Koopmanschap M: personal communication regarding data from Belgium and the UK, 1996

ESO Monographs
– Volumes already published in this series

F. Cavalli (Ed.)
Endocrine Therapy of Breast Cancer
Concepts and Strategies
VII, 120 pp.

J.F. Smyth (Ed.)
Interferons in Oncology
Current Status
and Future Directions
1987. VII, 70 pp.

F. Cavalli (Ed.)
Endocrine Therapy of Breast Cancer II
Current Developments and New
Methodologies
1987. VII, 65 pp.

L. Domellöf (Ed.)
Drug Delivery in Cancer Treatment
1987. VII, 99 pp.

L. Denis (Ed.)
The Medical Management of Prostate Cancer
1988. IX, 98 pp.

B. Winograd, M. Peckham,
H.M. Pinedo (Eds.)
Human Tumour Xenografts in Anticancer Drug Development
1988. XV, 143 pp. 37 figs.

A.B. Miller (Ed.)
Diet and the Aetiology of Cancer
1989. 2 figs. VII, 73 pages.

F. Cavalli (Ed.)
Endocrine Therapy of Breast Cancer III
1989. VII, 65 pp. 26 figs., 7 tabs.

L. Domellöf (Ed.)
Drug Delivery in Cancer Treatment II
Symptom Control, Cytokines,
Chemotherapy
1989. VII, 107 pp. 31 figs.

■ ■ ■ ■ ■ ■ ■ ■ ■ ■

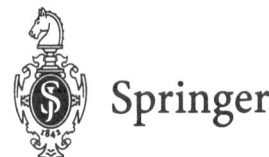

Springer

Springer-Verlag, P. O. Box 31 13 40, D-10643 Berlin, Germany

ESO Monographs
– Volumes already published in this series

A. Breit (Ed.)
**Magnetic Resonance
in Oncology**
1990. XIII, 173 pp. 147 figs., 7 tabs.

E.J. Freireich (Ed.)
**New Approaches to the
Treatment of Leukemia**
1990. VII, 193 pp. 37 figs., 36 tabs.

J.C. Holland, R. Zittoun (Eds.)
**Psychosocial Aspects
of Oncology**
1990. VIII, 142 pp. 3 figs.

L. Tomatis (Ed.)
**Air Pollution
and Human Cancer**
1990. VII, 86 pp. 7 figs., 10 tabs.

A. Goldhirsch (Ed.)
**Endocrine Therapy
of Breast Cancer IV**
1990. VII, 97 pp. 19 figs., 40 tabs.

R. Mertelsmann (Ed.)
**Lymphohaematopoietic
Growth Factors in Cancer
Therapy**
1990. VII, 90 pp. 8 figs., 14 tabs.

J. Hildebrand (Ed.)
**Neurological Adverse
Reactions to Anticancer
Drugs**
1990. VII, 99 pp. 8 figs., 15 tabs.

L. Domellöf (Ed.)
**Drug Delivery
in Cancer Treatment III**
Home Care – Symptom Control,
Economy, Brain Tumours
1990. VIII, 125 pp. 34 figs., 38 tabs.

S. Monfardini (Ed.)
**The Management of
Non-Hodgkin's Lymphomas
in Europe**
1990. VIII, 92 pp. 13 figs., 12 tabs.

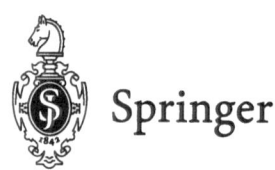

Springer-Verlag, P. O. Box 31 13 40, D-10643 Berlin, Germany

ESO Monographs
– Volumes already published in this series

L. Denis (Ed.)

**The Medical Management
of Prostate Cancer II**

1991. VII, 100 pp. 16 figs., 23 tabs.

A. Goldhirsch (Ed.)

**Endocrine Therapy
of Breast Cancer V**

1992. VIII, 103 pp. 33 figs. 20 tabs.

P.A. Bunn Jr. (Ed.)

**Current Topics
in Lung Cancer**

1991. VII, 82 pp. 1 fig., 24 tabs.

R. Mertelsmann (Ed.)

**Lymphohaematopoietic
Growth Factors in
CancerTherapy II**

1992. VII, 123 pp. 15 figs., 27 tabs.

D. Crowther (Ed.)

**Interferons:
Mechanisms of Action and
Role in Cancer Therapy**

1991. VII, 63 pp. 8 figs., 14 tabs.

P. Workman (Ed.)

**New Approaches in Cancer
Pharmacology: Drug Design
and Development**

1992. VII, 103 pp. 24 figs., 7 tabs.

W. Weber (Ed.)

Familial Cancer Control

1992. XIV, 126 pp. 29 figs., 29 tabs.

J. Hildebrand (Ed.)

**Management
in Neuro-Oncology**

1992. VII, 107 pp. 7 figs., 25 tabs.

M.B. Sporn (Ed.)

**Control of Growth Factors
and Prevention of Cancer**

1992. VIII, 74 pp. 22 figs., 4 tabs.

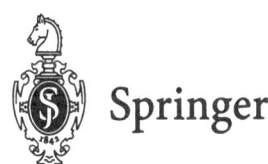

Springer

Springer-Verlag, P. O. Box 31 13 40, D-10643 Berlin, Germany

ESO Monographs
– Volumes already published in this series

A. Gad, M. Rosselli Del Turco (Eds.)
Breast Cancer Screening in Europe
1993. VIII, 148 pp. 25 figs., 39 tabs.

M.S. Aapro (Ed.)
Innovative Antimetabolites in Solid Tumours
1994. VII, 59 pp. 4 figs., 18 tabs.

L. Tomatis (Ed.)
Indoor and Outdoor Air Pollution and Human Cancer
1993. VII, 162 pp. 4 figs., 23 tabs.

P. Workman (Ed.)
New Approaches in Cancer Pharmacology: Drug Design and Development
Vol. II
1994. VII, 97 pp. 33 figs., 10 tabs.

K. Pummer (Ed.)
Biological Modulation of Solid Tumours by Interferons
1994. VII, 75 pp. 12 figs., 11 tabs.

– Currently available

A. Howell (Ed.)
Endocrine Therapy of Breast Cancer VI
1994. VII, 99 pp. 33 figs., 20 tabs.
Hardcover DM 96,-
ISBN 3-540-57690-8

L. Denis (Ed.)
Prostate Cancer 2000
1994. VII, 94 pp. 22 figs., 30 tabs.
Hardcover DM 108,-
ISBN 3-540-58296-7

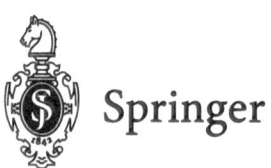

Springer

Springer-Verlag, P. O. Box 31 13 40, D-10643 Berlin, Germany

ESO Monographs
– Currently available

G.A. Pangalis (Ed.)
Malignant Lymphomas: Biology and Treatment
An Update
1995. IX, 189 pp. 29 figs., 47 tabs.
Hardcover DM 158,-
ISBN 3-540-60122-8

M. Tonato (Ed.)
Antiemetics in the Supportive Care of Cancer Patients
1996. VII, 145 pp. 3 figs., 28 tabs.
Hardcover DM 118,-
ISBN 3-540-61201-7

L. Degos, D.R. Parkinson (Eds.)
Retinoids in Oncology
1995. VII, 115 pp. 26 figs., 10 tabs.
Hardcover DM 118,-
ISBN 3-540-59181-8

L. Denis (Ed.)
Antiandrogens in Prostate Cancer
A Key to Tailored Endocrine Treatment
1996. VII, 120 pp. 54 figs., 39 tabs.
Hardcover DM 118,-
ISBN 3-540-60599-1

J.M. Dixon (Ed.)
Electropotentials in the Clinical Assessment of Breast Neoplasia
1996. VIII, 75 pp. 24 figs., 22 tabs.
Hardcover DM 82,-
ISBN 3-540-60348-4

Please order from
Springer-Verlag Berlin
Fax: + 49 / 30 / 8 27 87- 301
e-mail: orders@springer.de
or through your bookseller

Prices subject to change without notice.
In EU countries the local VAT is effec-

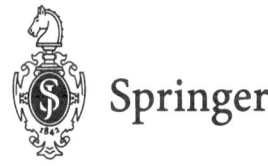

Springer

Springer-Verlag, P. O. Box 31 13 40, D-10643 Berlin, Germany

Springer
and the
environment

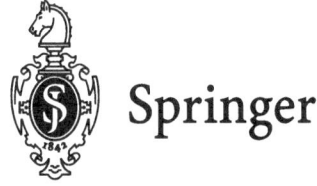 Springer